Take Time to Talk

Second Edition

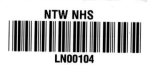

Take Time to Talk

Second Edition

A Resource for Apraxia Therapy, Esophageal Speech Training, Aphasia Therapy, and Articulation Therapy

Patricia F. White, M.A., CCC-SLP

Speech Pathologist, Rehabilitation Services

Department of Speech Pathology

Methodist Hospital Central

Memphis, Tennessee

Butterworth-Heinemann

Boston   Oxford   Johannesburg   Melbourne   New Dehli   Singapore

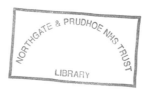

Library of Congress Cataloging-in-Publication Data
White, Patricia F., 1958-
    Take time to talk : a resource for apraxia therapy, esophageal speech training, aphasia therapy, and articulation therapy / Patricia F. White. -- 2nd ed.
        p.   cm.
    Includes bibliographical references.
    ISBN 0-7506-9783-0 (pbk. : alk. paper)
    1. Speech therapy--Exercises.   I. Title.
    [DNLM: 1. Speech Therapy--methods.   2. Speech Disorders--rehabilitation.   3. Speech, Esophageal.   4. Teaching Materials.
WL 340.2 W587t 1996]
RC423.W487   1996
616.85'506--dc20
DNLM/DLC
for Library of Congress   96-14174
                                                                              CIP

British Library Cataloguing-in-Publication Data
A catalogue record for this book is available from the British Library.

The publisher offers discounts on bulk orders of this book.
For information, please write:

Manager of Special Sales
Butterworth-Heinemann
313 Washington Street
Newton, MA 02158-1626
Tel: 617-928-2500
Fax: 617-928-2620

For information on all medical publications available, contact our World Wide Web home page at: http://www.bh.com/bh

10 9 8 7 6 5 4 3 2

Printed in the United States of America

This book is dedicated to Ann Stace Wood, Ph.D., my mentor and friend, who gave me my start in working with adult neurologically impaired patients, and to the many patients who have inspired its completion.

Contents

Preface

When I began my career in speech pathology over 13 years ago, I was lucky enough to find myself in a wonderful and diverse job setting. I completed my clinical fellowship year (CFY) by working in a private practice that contracted with an urban hospital, adult day care, and private school. My CFY supervisor was the first to spark my fascination in the disorder of apraxia and it was she that came up with the idea of my writing this workbook. With her encouragement I began to jot down on bits of paper all of the sentences and drills that were successful in helping my patients form words again and I added to the drills to meet their individual needs when a new problem or goal presented itself. As my experiences grew and I witnessed the success of the exercises, I developed a desire to share this information with other clinicians and patient families. Because there were no apraxia workbooks or resources on the market, I wanted to share what I felt was an important key in helping patients regain some meaningful form of communication.

The first edition of this book was printed in 1990. Since that time I have made numerous changes and revisions. Many of my patients have added their personal input to make it as practical and as useful as possible. I feel a deep debt of gratitude to those patients, for it was their ability to laugh in spite of a crippling disorder and offer words of encouragement that have greatly added to this book.

In this edition I have added more detailed instruction on how to use this book with patients, added more information on the disorders that this book was designed to help, and updated the references. When used creatively, this book is a valuable tool on a daily basis. It has withstood the test of time and has proven to be very useful for a number of disorders. I hope that you and your patients find it as enjoyable and beneficial as I have.

I wish to acknowledge my husband, Roger N. White, who spent many hours helping me format this book and without whose help this book would not have been completed.

Patricia F. White

HOW TO USE THIS BOOK WITH APRAXIC PATIENTS

Take Time to Talk is a step-by-step instructional guide for verbally apraxic patients. It is based on a traditional apraxia approach as described in *Language Intervention Strategies in Adult Aphasia* by Roberta Chapey (Williams and Wilkins Publishers, 1986) and in *Motor Speech Disorders: Substrates, Differential Diagnosis, and Management* by J. R. Duffy (Mosby Year Book, 1995). The text is arranged in alphabetical order for convenience. Each exercise progresses from easier productions to more difficult ones to provide a challenge for all levels of apraxia. The last sounds of the words are arranged in the order that they would emerge in child language. Since most apraxic patients also have an aphasic component, a picture stimulus may be required to help them conceptualize the word. For this reason several pictures have been included for each sound.

It is essential to begin with a good evaluation and a proper diagnosis. Remember, just because a patient cannot repeat words and phrases does not always indicate an apraxia. Patients with Wernicke's aphasia and conduction aphasia also have trouble with verbal repeating tasks. A good resource for your evaluation can be found in *Apraxia of Speech in Adults: The Disorder and Its Management* by Wertz, LaPointe, and Rosenbek (Singular Publishing Group, Inc., 1991).

Apraxic patients need visual as well as auditory cueing. Very severely apraxic patients may require a picture cue, a written cue, an auditory cue, and a visual cue. The cues should be diminished as they progress through therapy in order to increase their volitional control. You will want to drop off one method of cueing at a time.

CHARACTERISTICS OF PATIENTS WITH APRAXIA

1. They struggle to untangle their words
2. Their initial phonemes are more in error than their final phonemes.
3. They have inconsistent errors.
4. Their involuntary speech is better than their voluntary.
5. Their errors are of substitution, repetition, omission, and distortion.
6. Their errors increase with word complexity.
7. Their errors increase as the words increase in length.
8. Visual cues help them.
9. They are aware of their errors.
10. Their consonant productions are usually more in error than their vowel productions.
11. They have better accuracy for meaningful utterances than for non-meaningful ones.

Therapy using the picture drills might follow this format:

CLINICIAN: Using the page with the picture cues and printed words, the clinician points to a picture and provides a stimulus sentence, e.g., "Row, row, row your boat."

CLINICIAN: Says the sentence cue again, pausing before the target word to allow the patient to complete the sentence, e.g., "Row, row, row your _____."

PATIENT: Completes the sentence. "Boat"

CLINICIAN: Repeats target utterance. "Boat"

PATIENT: Repeats target utterance. "Boat"

CLINICIAN: Mouths the target utterance, removing the auditory cue, but still providing the visual cue.

PATIENT: Repeats target utterance aloud. "Boat"

CLINICIAN: Allows for a 3 to 5 second delay and then asks the patient, "What did you say?"

PATIENT: Repeats the utterance. "Boat"

CLINICIAN: Turns to the page with the pictures without the printed word, removing the printed word cue and repeats the same steps.

Therapy using the fill-in sentence drills might follow this format:

CLINICIAN: Says the fill-in sentence cue completely, e.g., "The opposite of girl is boy."

CLINICIAN: Says the fill-in sentence cue pausing before the target word to allow the patient to complete the sentence, e.g., "The opposite of girl is _____."

PATIENT: Completes the sentence. "Boy"

CLINICIAN: Repeats target utterance. "Boy"

PATIENT: Repeats target utterance. "Boy"

CLINICIAN: Mouths the target utterance, removing the auditory cue, but still providing the visual cue.

PATIENT: Repeats target utterance aloud. "Boy"

CLINICIAN: Allows for a 3 to 5 second delay and then asks the patient, "What did you say?"

PATIENT: Repeats the utterance. "Boy"

Therapy using the single syllable words, two-word and three-word phrases, and question drills might follow this format:

CLINICIAN: Says the target utterance. "Big ball"

PATIENT: Repeats the target utterance. "Big ball"

CLINICIAN: Asks the patient to repeat the target utterance 3 times in a row. The clinician will say the utterance with the patient on the first try, mouth the utterance taking away the auditory cue on the second try, and does nothing as the patient says the utterance the third time, taking away the visual cue.

PATIENT: Says the target utterance 3 times in a row. "Big ball, big ball, big ball"

CLINICIAN: Allows for a 3 to 5 second delay and then asks, "What did you just say?"

PATIENT: Says the target utterance again. "Big ball"

It is important to have the patient repeat each stimulus word several times. You will know your patient best and the appropriate level at which to begin. I have found that some of the easiest sounds to begin with are /b/, /m/, /p/, and /w/.

Depending on the severity of the apraxia, therapy might follow this progression:

1. Blowing out a match. Blowing bubbles. Creating a fog on a mirror. Eliciting "ah" by role-playing a doctor checking the patient's throat using a tongue depressor, etc.
2. Automatic speech tasks, such as singing familiar songs, counting, saying the days of the week, prayers, nursery rhymes, etc.
3. Repeating syllables.
4. Reading syllables.
5. Filling in a word at the end of a sentence.
6. Repeating words after the therapist.
7. Repeating words heard on a tape recorder.
8. Reading single words from a word list.
9. Filling in two words at the end of a sentence.
10. Repeating two-word phrases after the therapist.
11. Reading two-word phrases.
12. Repeating three-word phrases.
13. Reading three-word phrases.
14. Answering a question with a word.
15. Answering conversational questions.
16. Role-playing.

FAMILIAR SONGS WITH REPETITIVE LYRICS

Merrily We Roll Along
Happy Birthday
For He's a Jolly Good Fellow
London Bridge
Mary Had a Little Lamb
Good Night, Ladies!
Jesus Loves Me
Jacob's Ladder
Good Morning to You
My Bonnie Lies Over the Ocean
Row, Row, Row Your Boat
Michael, Row Your Boat Ashore
Ten Little Indians
Deep and Wide
I've Got the Joy, Joy, Joy, Joy (Down in My Heart)
Oh, Dear, What Can the Matter Be?
Oh Won't You Sit Down?
O Christmas Tree
Where Has My Little Dog Gone?
What Do You Do with a Drunken Sailor?
Jimmy Cracked Corn
My Darling Clementine
He's Got the Whole World in His Hands
The Old Gray Mare
She'll Be Comin' Round the Mountain
When the Saints Go Marching In
We Wish You a Merry Christmas
Do, Lord, Remember Me

NOTE: Sing these songs at half speed to allow your patient to sing along with you.

HELPFUL SUGGESTIONS

Have your patient watch your mouth as you say the words for visual cueing.

Present the stimulus words in a rhythmic manner or a "sing-song" fashion.

Practice their successes not their failures.

Be creative. Create your own carrier phrases that are meaningful to your patient.

Keep frustration to a minimum.

Pair the target word with its symbolic gesture, for example, waving hello and good-bye.

Work on one sound at a time until it is firmly established. In this manner, another sound may be more easily added. For example, establish /b/, and then add /m/ or /w/ words.

It is very important to have consistent, frequent practice. Short frequent sessions are better than long infrequent sessions. For this reason, it is a good idea to train a family member or friend to work with the patient to insure that the patient practices several times a day.

If working on multisyllabic words, break them up into syllables and print them for the patient to read (for example, choc - o - late or pi - an - o).

If your patient has good reading comprehension, have a written description of how the sounds are formed (for example, /f/ is formed by biting your bottom lip, /b/ is formed by blotting your lips and turning on the voice box).

CASE ILLUSTRATION:

One of my favorite patients was a sixty-nine year-old woman who was rendered nonverbal following a stroke. Her diagnosis was severe oral-verbal apraxia mixed with expressive aphasia, severe agraphia, and mild receptive aphasia. When therapy began, she was only able to produce grunts, groans, and an occasional "oh." She could not imitate any oral motor movements. She would struggle to blow out a match. Her attempts at vowel imitations were unsuccessful and she was unable to sing any familiar songs. She would pull and tug at her mouth in a desperate attempt to form words.

We continued to try to elicit language through the use of singing repetitive tunes. She was occasionally able to manage to sing a word or two at the end of the lyrics. I began singing lines from songs having an /m/ word at the end of the line, for example, "By the light of the silvery moon," "Three blind mice," and "Daniel Boone was a man." She was able to sing the last word of these lines with me. These were the only three words she could produce for a couple of sessions. She simply could not produce a word without the musical melody.

Gradually we were able to faze out the melodies and she began to produce those three words with just the spoken fill-in sentence cue. After this breakthrough we were able to slowly add other /m/ words using the fill-in sentence cues. We worked on adding other bilabial consonants in the same way over a period of several months. By that time the other sounds were coming much easier. At the end of several months of very systematic therapy she was able to converse in slow halting sentences.

5

HOW TO USE THIS BOOK WITH LARYNGECTOMEES

This book can be used in teaching esophageal speech by using the consonant injection method. Esophageal speech is made by injecting or pushing air into the upper esophagus and then immediately releasing it to produce a belching sound. Patients can learn to control this sound to form speech.

Most esophageal speakers are able to produce some spontaneous esophageal sound in connected speech. Often they are unaware of the way in which the sound was produced. They are using the voiceless sounds in speech to push air into their esophagus. By having the patient read or repeat the voiceless sound words and phrases in this book, you can help him form his new voice. For example, have the patient repeat a phrase, such as "tic-tac-toe", again and again until he begins to produce esophageal sound. Have the patient press the tip of his tongue hard against his hard palate. See if the patient can feel a small bubble of air trapped between his tongue and his hard palate. Ask the patient to try to push the ball of air into his throat as he reads from the /t/ two- and three-word phrase list. As the patient reads the /t/ words the tongue will be in position to inject air into the esophageal space.

You can use the /t/, /tʃ/, /s/, /k/, and /p/ words and phrases in teaching the consonant injection method. The words and phrases upon which the patient has early success should be repeated over and over until the patient can produce esophageal sound each time he tries. The words and phrases upon which he has success can later be used as carrier phrases for the more difficult sounds.

NOTE: Before esophageal speech training is ever attempted, an insufflation test should be performed on the patient to see if he is physically capable of producing esophageal sound.

CASE ILLUSTRATION

I was working with a fifty-five year-old woman who had had a recent laryngectomy. During the first few sessions we were focusing on the mechanics of esophageal speech production. I instructed her to press her tongue firmly against the roof of her mouth to trap air between her tongue and hard palate and with her mouth closed to pump with the back of the tongue to force the air into her esophagus. My descriptions, illustrations, and demonstrations were not having any success, and she was growing frustrated. I noticed in our conversations that she was able to spontaneously produce some esophageal sound. Further observation of her speech revealed that all of her spontaneous speech productions were on words beginning with the /t/ sound. We stopped focusing on the mechanics of esophageal speech production and began to work exclusively from the /t/ word list. She had almost 100% production on the /t/ words. She began to relax and enjoy her new voice. After her "spontaneous" success with /t/ words she was able to realize how she was producing the esophageal sound. She quickly became quite accomplished with her new voice. She returned to work after two to three months more of therapy and became the new president of the local Lost Chord Club.

HOW TO USE THIS BOOK WITH APHASIC PATIENTS

This book can easily be adapted to be used with patients who have aphasia.

1. The picture pages can be used in auditory comprehension tasks for picture identification.
2. The picture pages can also be used for low-level writing tasks where the patient is asked to copy each word. Turn to the page without the written words and have the patient try to write each word under the pictures.
3. The fill-in sentence pages are helpful with patients who have anomia.
4. The question pages can be used for auditory comprehension tasks.
5. The question pages can be used for reading comprehension tasks.
6. Page 159 can be used for categorical naming with high-level aphasics.

HOW TO USE THIS BOOK WITH DYSARTHIC PATIENTS

The words and phrases can be used to strengthen muscles weakened by a stroke. The /k/ and /g/ sections can be used to exercise the posterior tongue and the /t/, /d/, /n/, and /l/ can be used to exercise the tongue tip. You can target the sounds that your patients have the most difficulty producing.

CHARACTERISTICS OF PATIENTS WITH DYSARTHRIA

1. The muscles of respiration, articulation, phonation, resonation, and/or prosody may be affected.
2. Their articulation errors are consistent.
3. Their articulation errors are of simplification and distortion.
4. They simplify consonant clusters.
5. Their speech is slurred.
6. Their intelligibility is usually improved if they use a slower rate of speech.

HELPFUL SUGGESTIONS

It is very important to have consistent, frequent practice. Short frequent sessions are better than long infrequent sessions. For this reason, it is a good idea to train a family member or friend to work with the patient to insure he/she practices several times a day.

Have your patient exaggerate the articulation movements as he/she says each word.

Have your patient practice slowing his/her rate of speech. Speed is not the objective; increased intelligibility is.

Work on words that are significant to your patient, e.g., family members' names, pets' names, etc.

HOW TO USE THIS BOOK WITH CHILDREN

This book is easily adapted to use in therapy with children who have articulation errors or phonological processing problems.

1. The word lists and picture pages provide a resource for initial consonant production to be used in speech tasks.
2. An extra section has been provided as a resource for final consonants. It is located at the back of this workbook.
3. This workbook provides a resource for deep testing consonant productions.
4. The /h/ exercises can be used for easy onset drills with patients who have vocal hyperfunction disorders, such as, vocal nodules.

SUGGESTED READINGS

Chapey, R. *Language Intervention Strategies in Adult Aphasia, Second Edition.* Baltimore: Williams and Wilkins Publishers, 1986, 420-432.

Darley, F.L., Aronson, A.E., and Brown, J.R. *Motor Speech Disorders.* Philadelphia: W. B. Saunders Company, 1975, 86-98, 250-269.

Duffy, J.R. *Motor Speech Disorders: Substrates, Differential Diagnosis and Management.* St. Louis: Mosby Year Book, 1995, 417-431.

Dworkin, J.P. *Motor Speech Disorders: A Treatment Guide.* St. Louis: Mosby Year Book, 1991, 32-38.

Johns, D.F. *Clinical Management of Neurologic Communicative Disorders.* Boston: Little, Brown, and Company, 1978, 191-238.

Lauder, E. *Self-Help for the Laryngectomee.* 11115 Whisper Hollow, San Antonio, Texas, 1979.

Marquardt, T. and Cannito, M. Treatment of Verbal Apraxia in Broca's Aphasia. In Wallace, G. (eds.). *Adult Aphasia Rehabilitation.* Boston: Butterworth-Heinemann, 1996.

Vogel, D. and Cannito, M. *Treating Disordered Speech Motor Control: For Clinicians by Clinicians.* Austin: Pro-Ed, Inc., 1991.

Wertz, R.T., LaPointe, L., and Rosenbek, J.C. *Apraxia of Speech in Adults: The Disorder and Its Management.* San Diego: Singular Publishing Group, Inc., 1991.

The B Sound

The opposite of girl is _____.	boy
I was stung by a bumble _____.	bee
All work and no play makes Jack a dull _____.	boy
Tie the ribbon in a _____.	bow
When you leave, you say good- _____.	bye
I'm as busy as a _____.	bee
I got up on the wrong side of the _____.	bed
You get in a tub to take a _____.	bath
You sleep in a _____.	bed
You hit a ball with a _____.	bat
Ring the _____.	bell
You sail in a sail _____.	boat
He couldn't hit the broad side of a _____.	barn
The opposite of good is _____.	bad
If you don't have a car you ride on a _____.	bus
I'm as hungry as a _____.	bear
I put my money in a _____.	bank
The opposite of front is _____.	back
When a man loses his hair, he is _____.	bald
The opposite of little is _____.	big
A male cow is a _____.	bull
A mouse is little; an elephant is _____.	big
The runner was tagged at third _____.	base
I let the cat out of the _____.	bag
Row, row, row your _____.	boat

11

His bark is worse than his _____.	bite
A bird in the hand is worth two in the _____.	bush
A blue jay and a sparrow are two kinds of _____.	birds
A watched pot never _____.	boils
A barking dog never _____.	bites
He who laughs last, laughs _____.	best
To end World War II, the U.S.A. dropped the atom _____.	bomb
Abraham Lincoln was killed by John Wilkes _____.	Booth
Another name for infant is _____.	baby
For breakfast I had eggs and _____.	bacon
The opposite of above is _____.	below
Don't put all your eggs in one _____.	basket

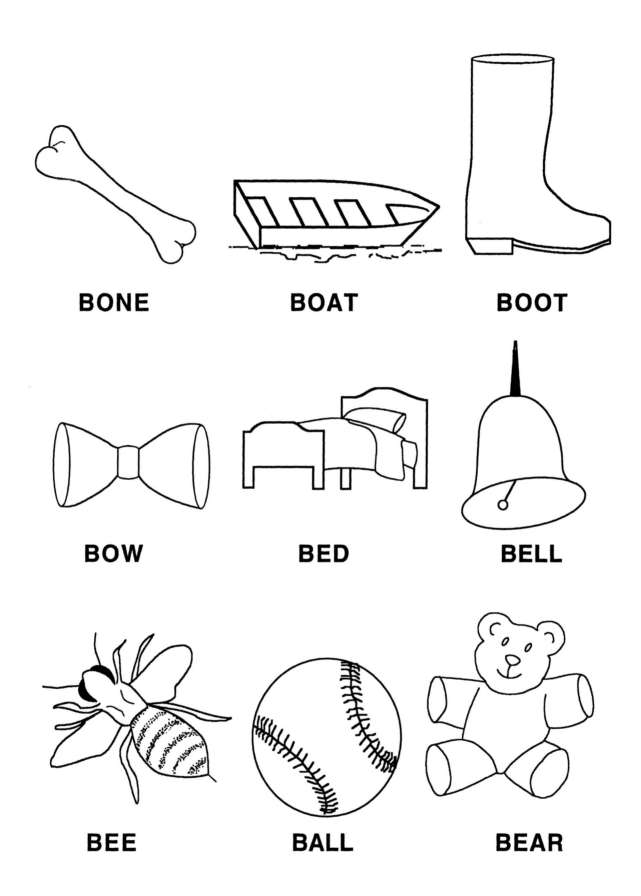

BONE   **BOAT**   **BOOT**

BOW   **BED**   **BELL**

BEE   **BALL**   **BEAR**

13

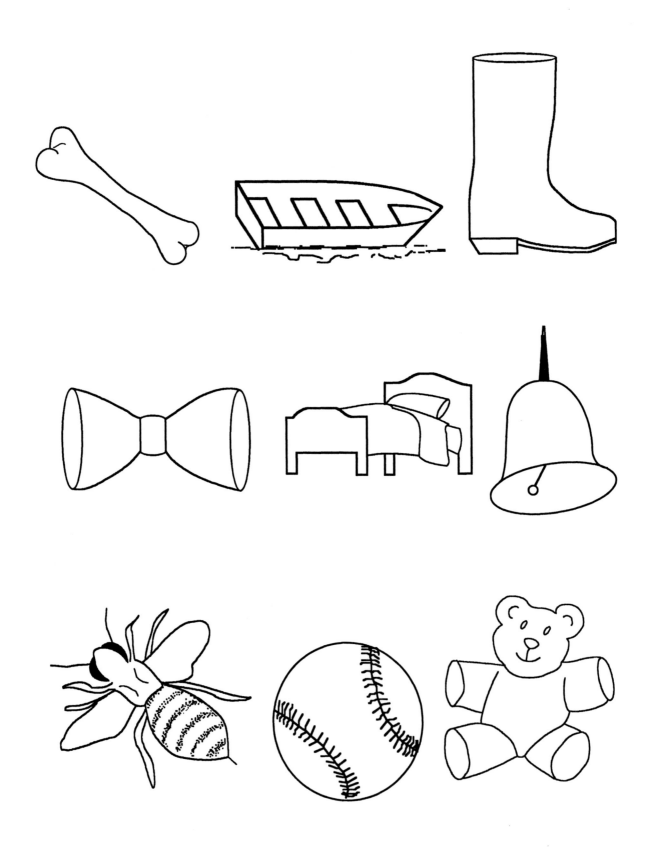

14

bay	bag	boil
be, bee	beg	bowl
by, bye	big	bull
beau, bow	bug	bear, bare
bow	bad	bar
boo	bead	beer
boy	bed	bore
bop	bid	bur
beep	bud	base, bass
beam	bait	bass
bomb	bat	bus
boom	bet	boss
bum	beat, beet	beach, beech
ban	bit	bush
been, bin	bite	bash
Ben	bout	buzz
bone	boot	booze
bun	but, butt	beige
bean	boat	bath
bib	bang	Beth
bob, Bob	buff	both
babe	beef	booth
back	ball, bawl	bathe
bake	bail, bale	balk
beak	bell, belle	bulk
book	bile	bald
buck	bill, Bill	bold

build	box
balm	beard
band	bird
bend	board
bind	belch
bound	bench
bank	bunch
bunk	berth, birth
bark	belt
barn	bolt
born	built
burn	bent
bask	bunt
barge	birch
badge	bisque
barb	bond
baste	bounce
beast	bowl
best	bulb
boast	bulge
boost	bump
burst	Butch

buy back	bell-bottoms
bellboy	beer bottle
big boy	beer barrel
big ball	ball bearing
big boat	big balloon
big bucks	best buddy
bedbug	burned bacon
barbell	baby bed
bad boy	baby bird
bad book	busy bee
baseball	bubble bath
backbone	beetle bug
bankbook	butter bean
bunk bed	buzzing bee
bird book	basketball
bird beak	bowling ball
bail bond	busybody
backbite	baby bottle
bareback	baby buggy
boy's band	baby bonnet
birdbath	busy beaver
backboard	belly button
buckboard	bathing beauty
baked beans	banana boat
build a barn	

17

Bob bit Bill.

big bed bugs

baseball bat

big bad boy

Bill buys boats.

best built boat

burned baked beans

Bob built a barn.

Boston boy's band

Boston baked beans

big balloons burst

busy beetle bug

bouncing baby boy

bouncing bowling ball

The beans began to boil.

Bob began to be bossy.

Bill bought a bird bath.

Buy a better built boat.

Buy the big bird book.

Betty burned the baked beans.

Bart is a big bad boy.

Bob begged Betty to bake.

Bill bought the best boat.

Buddy bought a baseball bat.

Which is bigger, a bird or an ant?

Which can you ride, a bike or a cup?

Which is wilder, a bear or a pony?

Which goes around your waist, a belt or a sock?

Which is alive, a bee or a bed?

Which is painful, a burn or a hug?

Which is younger, a man or a boy?

Which will ring, a bell or a pencil?

Which is more expensive, a sheet or a bed?

Which is round, a ball or a phone?

Which is meat, an apple or bacon?

Do you read a book or a chair?

Which can fly, a bird or a dog?

Which will float, a car or a boat?

Do you sleep in a bed or a sink?

Which business handles your money, a bank or a post office?

Which can sting, a butterfly or a bee?

Which is bigger, a bear or a mouse?

Which is younger, a teen or a baby?

Which is a male, a bull or a cow?

Which will roll, a ball or a book?

Which is a vegetable, beans or bananas?

Do you drink beer or cereal?

Which do you put on toast, chalk or butter?

Which one is round, a football or a baseball?

Which one carries more people, a bus or a car?

Which goes on your foot, a boot or a hat?

blue	blaze	brook
blow	blouse	brag
blip	blink	brig
blame	blank	brad, Brad
bloom	blanch	braid
blown	bland	bread, bred
blab	blind	breed
blob	blond	bride
black	blast	broad
bleak	blest	brood
block	blimp	bright
bloke	blunt	brute
blade	blurb	bring
bleed	blurt	brief
bled	brew	brawl
blood	brow	broil
bleat	bream	Braille
blight	brim	brace
bloat	broom	brass
blot	brain	Bruce
bluff	bran	breech, breach
blare	brown	brooch, broach
blur	brawn	brush
bless	bribe	brash
bliss	brake, break	braze, braise
bleach	brick	bruise
blush	broke	breeze

brave
breath
broth
breathe
branch
brand
breast
bridge
brink
brisk
bronze
brunt

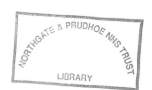

The Ch Sound

He bit off more than he could _____.	chew
The criminal had to wear a ball and _____.	chain
Rats like to eat cheddar _____.	cheese
The opposite of expensive is _____.	cheap
On Sunday we go worship at a _____.	church
It is better to turn the other _____.	cheek
A baby chicken is called a _____.	chick
The leader of an Indian tribe is called a _____.	chief
Tell someone and get it off your _____.	chest
We went on a wild goose _____.	chase
The murderer was sent to the electric _____.	chair
The bank would not cash my _____.	check
Butter was once made in a _____.	churn
Peking is the capital of _____.	China
Beggars can't be _____.	choosers
Life is just a bowl of _____.	cherries
He's as young as a spring _____.	chicken

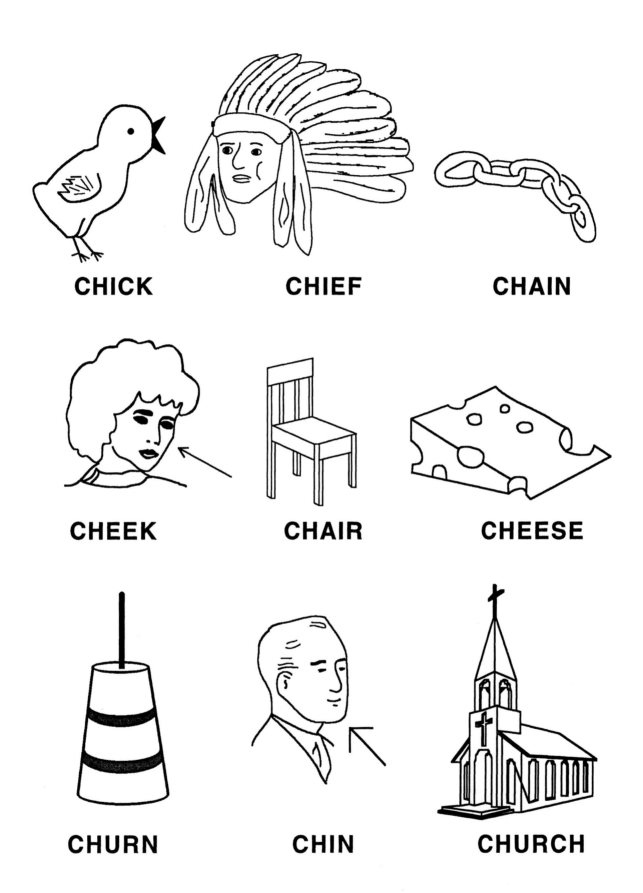

CHICK   CHIEF   CHAIN

CHEEK   CHAIR   CHEESE

CHURN   CHIN   CHURCH

23

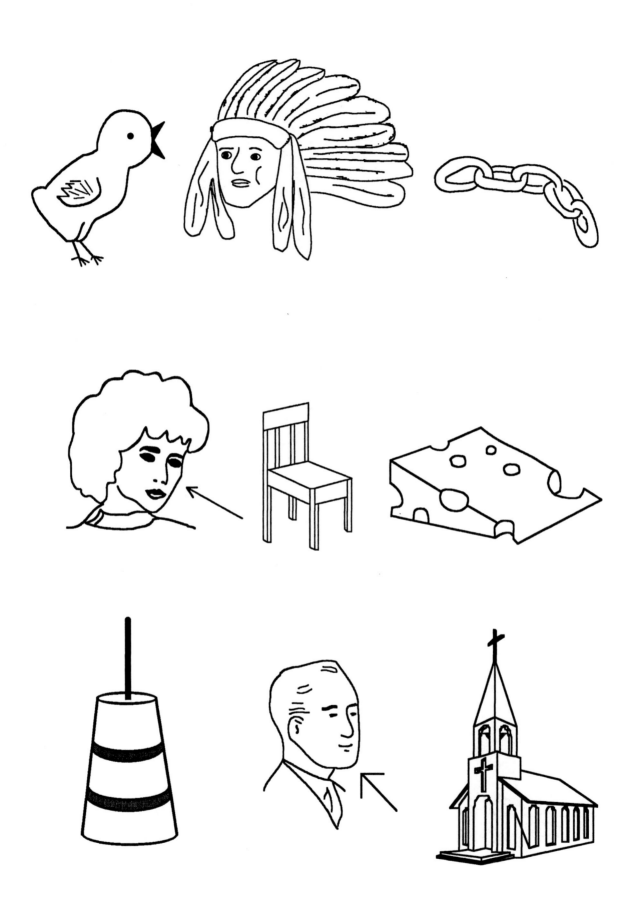

24

chew	cheer
chow	chore
chap	chase
cheap, cheep	chess
chip	choice
chop	church
chime	cheese
chum	chose
chain	choose
chin	chive
check	champ
cheek	chimp
chick	chomp
choke	chance
chuck	change
chug	charge
Chad	charm
chide	chart
chit	chaste
cheat	chalk
chat	chaps
chafe	chant
chaff	chest
chief	chirp
chill	child
chair	chump
char	churn

cha-cha

chowchow

choo choo

chitchat

cheap chair

chess champ

chump change

church chapel

church chancel

change channels

charred chicken

chess and checkers

chilly church

chunky cheese

cheddar cheese

chubby cheeks

Charlie Chan

chipped china

chilly chapel

chopped chicken

Chinese checkers

Chubby Checkers

chubby children

chipper chipmunks

charming children

chocolate chip

Cherokee chief

chilly church chapel

charming chubby child

chunky chocolate chips

chess and checkers
   champ

Charlie changed the
   channel.

Is bubble gum expensive or cheap?

Which is part of the face, the elbow or the chin?

Which is a baby, a chicken or a chick?

Which is the leader, the chief or the Indian?

Is Swiss a type of cheese or flower?

Is the winner the loser or the champ?

Does a shirt cover your chest or legs?

Would you find an altar in a school or a church?

Does a bird chirp or bark?

Was butter made in a churn or a kettle?

Which is a board game, golf or chess?

Do you write with thread or chalk?

Do you sit on a chair or a table?

Is it wrong to give or cheat?

Which is a substitute for money, a check or an ad?

Do whiskers grow on your arm or your chin?

Does an ax paint or chop?

Is February hot or chilly?

Is it painful to smile or choke?

Do bells chime or sing?

Do your teeth help you chew or think?

Which is stronger, a string or a chain?

Is a two year old an adult or a child?

Do cowboys wear dresses or chaps?

Is Peking in China or Italy?

Do more children play bridge or chase?

The D Sound

They are as different as night and _____.	day
A female deer is called a _____.	doe
Give credit where credit is _____.	due
The opposite of live is _____.	die
I have a mom and a _____.	dad
The opposite of alive is _____.	dead
Helen Keller was blind, deaf, and _____.	dumb
The opposite of shallow is _____.	deep
A German Shepherd is a kind of _____.	dog
When you leave, please close the _____.	door
The opposite of up is _____.	down
The opposite of light is _____.	dark
It's always darkest before the _____.	dawn
Five cents is a nickel; ten cents is a _____.	dime
The opposite of sharp is _____.	dull
That is easier said than _____.	done
You use a shovel to _____.	dig
Beauty is only skin _____.	deep
What goes up, must come _____.	down
It's raining cats and _____.	dogs
What's up _____?	doc
He bet it all on one roll of the _____.	dice
Give me liberty or give me _____.	death
Pretty is as pretty _____.	does
The opposite of clean is _____.	dirty

28

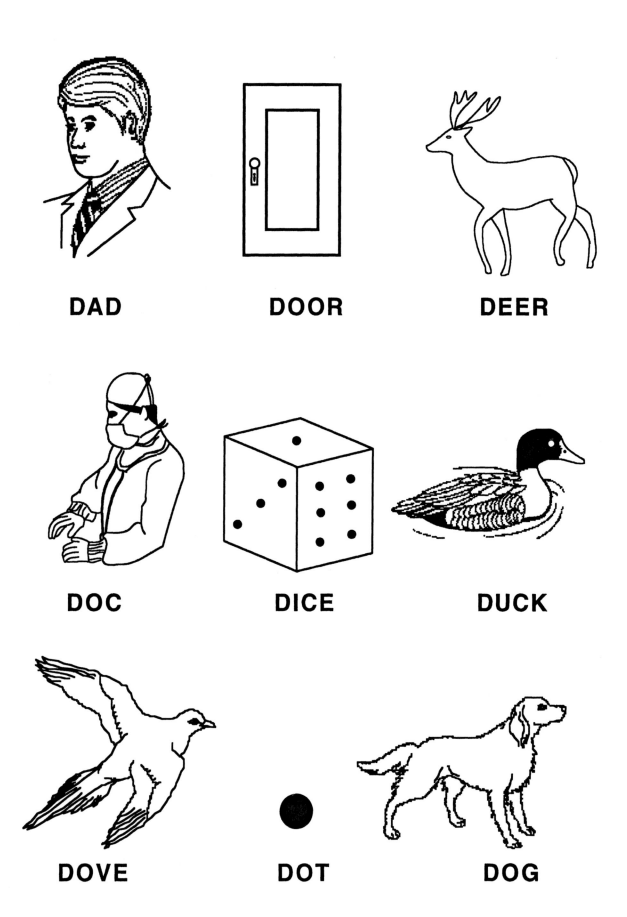

DAD **DOOR** **DEER**

DOC **DICE** **DUCK**

DOVE **DOT** **DOG**

29

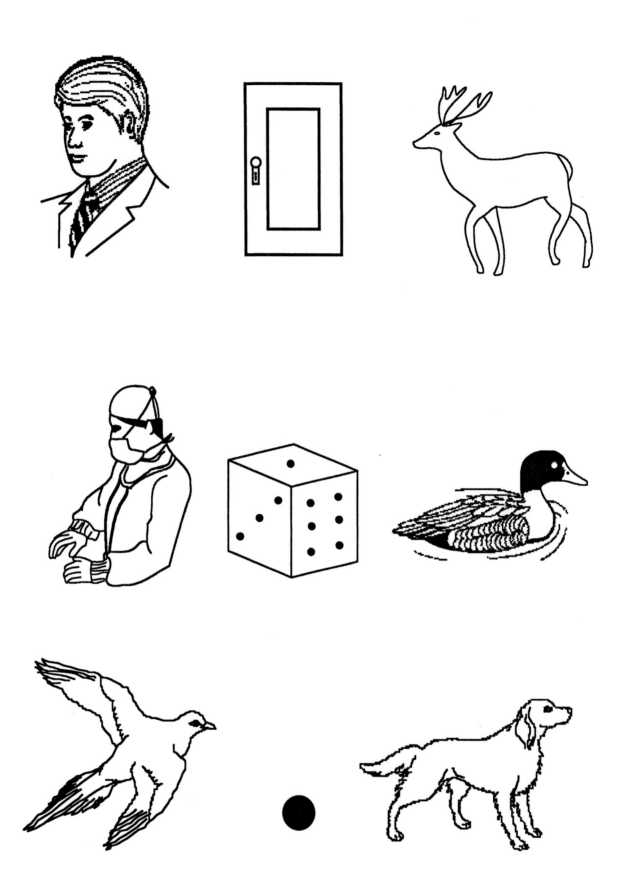

day	daub	dial
die, dye	deck	dill
do, dew, due	duke	dole
doe, dough	dike	doll
deep	dock, Doc	dull
dip	duck	dell
dope	dug, Doug	dare
dame	dig	deer, dear
dam, damn	dog	dire
deem	dude	door
dim	Dad	deuce
dime	dead	dice
dome	deed	dose
doom	died	douse, dowse
dumb	did	dace
Dan	dud	dish
den	dote	dash
dean, Dean	date	doze
dawn	debt	daze
dine	dot	does
dune	ding	Dave
down	dong	dove
done	duff	dive
Don	deaf	death
deign	doff	damp
dub	dale	dump
dab	deal	dance

dense
dunce
dark
darn
dank
dunk
dart
dirt
dealt
deft
dent
depth
desk
disk, disc
dusk
ditch
Dutch
don't
dodge
duct
dust

doodad

due date

dig deep

die down

deep dish

dead duck

ding-dong

dive deep

duck down

dark day

doomsday

deaf and dumb

dime a dozen

dig ditches

daredevil

death defying

dirty dog

dirty deal

decoy duck

Dandy Dan

Daffy Duck

Donald Duck

double-deal

double dose

double date

dinner date

dillydally

daily double

dirty dishes

double-decker

daily diary

dental decay

Daddy's darling

Duck down, Dan.

Don't die down.

dark damp day

dig deep ditches

Don's dirty dog

Don't dillydally.

Dad's deaf and dumb.

Do the dirty dishes.

dirty double-deal

divers delve deep

Dad's darling daughter

Dan is a dead duck.

Debbie doesn't do dishes.

Daredevils are death
   defying.

33

Which is bigger, a mouse or a dog?

Which one can quack, a duck or a cat?

Which is a female, a doe or a buck?

Which can fly, a dove or a dog?

Which is worth ten cents, a dime or a quarter?

Which is male, your dad or your mom?

When is the sun out, night or day?

Which is a toy, a doll or a chair?

Is a well shallow or deep?

Which is in the morning, dawn or sunset?

When you use a shovel, do you dig or saw?

Do you walk out a door or a window?

When you buy a house, do you get a lease or a deed?

Which is faster, a deer or a cat?

If you can't hear, are you deaf or lame?

If you can't talk, are you blind or dumb?

Is the ocean shallow or deep?

Which is a boy's name, Debbie or Dean?

Is the Hoover a dam or a bridge?

Is a mallard a dog or a duck?

Is George Washington alive or dead?

Does a phone have a knob or a dial?

Is the Tango a dance or a game?

Is night light or dark?

Does gravity pull things up or down?

Do you play craps with cards or dice?

draw	drug
dry	dread
dray	drill
drew	droll
drape	drool
drip	dress
droop	dross
drop	drowse
dream	drive
drum	drove
drain	draft
drone	drift
drown	drink
drawn	drank
drab	drunk
drake	dredge
drag	

The F Sound

The opposite of many is _____.	few
Put another log on the _____.	fire
The opposite of skinny is _____.	fat
Another name for autumn is _____.	fall
The opposite of near is _____.	far
Old Mac Donald had a _____.	farm
The opposite of slow is _____.	fast
You wear shoes on your _____.	feet
Look in the lost and _____.	found
The opposite of empty is _____.	full
The opposite of last is _____.	first
The number after three is _____.	four
Only you can prevent forest _____.	fires
There are twelve inches in a _____.	foot
Let's go fishing and catch a few _____.	fish
The number after four is _____.	five
The eyes, nose, and mouth are all part of the _____.	face
A baby deer is called a _____.	fawn
Minks are raised for their _____.	fur
The opposite of true is _____.	false
The grass is always greener on the other side of the _____.	fence
He is as sly as a _____.	fox
I have a mother and a _____.	father
Absence makes the heart grow _____.	fonder
You wear a ring on your _____.	finger

36

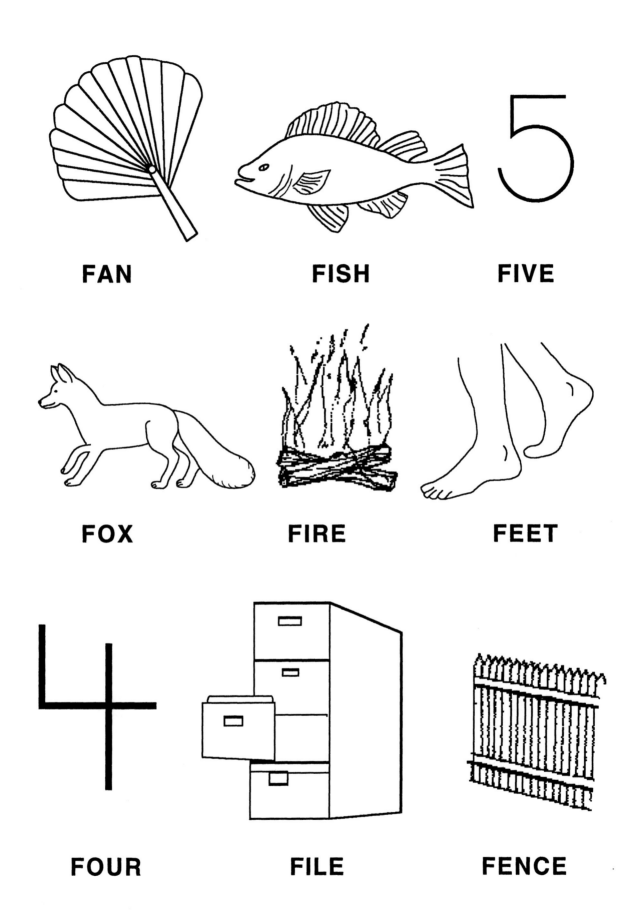

FAN   FISH   FIVE

FOX   FIRE   FEET

FOUR   FILE   FENCE

37

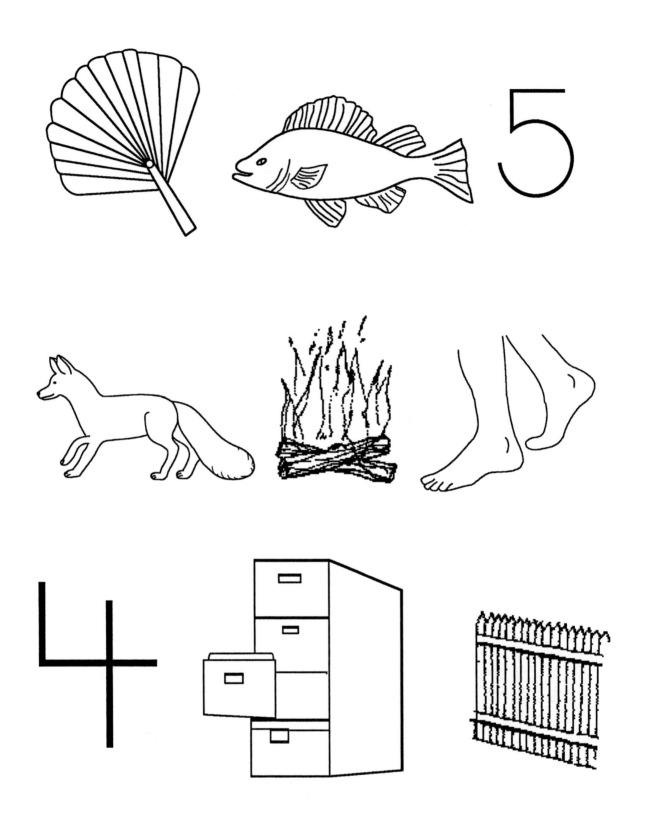

38

fee	fat	fish
fey, Faye	fate	faze, phase
foe	feet, feat	fuzz
few	fit	fuse
fie	fight	fizz
fop	foot	five
fame	fang	faith
foam	fife	false
fume	fail	fact
fan	fall	farm
fawn	file	firm
phone	fill, Phil	form
fine	foil	fast
fin	full	feast
feign, fain	foul, fowl	fault
fun	feel	felt
fib	fool	faint
fob	fell	fount
fake	fuel	fend
fig	for, four, fore	fiend
fog	fir, fur	find
fad	fire	fond
fed	far	found
feed	fair, fare	fund
fade	fear	fern
feud	face	fetch
food	fuss	field

fold

fierce

force

fifth

film

filth

finch

first

fix

fox

folk

ford

forge

fork

fort

forth, fourth

fudge

furl

feel fit

fish fin

feel fine

fivefold

fish food

four fish

face facts

fox fur

fist fight

face first

farm fowl

force field

find fault

fierce fight

fuss and fume

farfetched

firefighter

fat fellow

forefather

five fingers

forefinger

fish fillet

first family

forty-four

forty-five

fifty-four

fifty-five

funny face

funny farm

finger food

football fan

finish first

fifty-fifty

foster family

family photo

photo finish

fiddle-faddle

facial feature

fine fox fur

four fat fish

fall face first

force-feed food

fierce fist fight

foes fuss and fight

five fat fingers

first fix the faucet

five feeble fingers

five funny faces

Faye found a football.

fifty-five fish

fancy fantail fish

fifty-five fat fellows

forty-four fat fish

Phil found a family photo.

Is October in the spring or the fall?

Is a cow found in the city or on a farm?

Which lives in the water, a fox or a fish?

Do you wear a ring on your finger or your leg?

Are your eyes on your face or feet?

Is your mother a male or female?

Do you wear shoes on your hands or feet?

Which is hotter, fire or ice?

Is a jet slow or fast?

Which is longer, a foot or an inch?

Which is lighter, a feather or a rock?

Which is a baby deer, a colt or a fawn?

How many fingers are on each hand, four or five?

Is a counterfeit real or fake?

Is a blue jay a fowl or a fish?

Is a flounder a fish or an insect?

Does a fish have wings or fins?

Do restaurants serve food or clothes?

Which is a smaller number, five or ten?

Which one is wilder, a cat or a fox?

Is gasoline a food or a fuel?

Is your enemy your foe or your friend?

Is a lie the truth or a fib?

Is the sun near or far?

Do you eat peas with a fork or a knife?

Was the Alamo a fort or a castle?

Is the truth fact or fiction?

fly	flute	frown
flaw	fling	freak
flay	fluff	frock
flea, flee	flail	frog
flow	flair, flare	fried
flew, flu	flier	fraud
flap	floor	fright
flip	floss	freight
flop	fleece	fret
flame	flash	fruit
flume	flesh	frail
flab	flush	frill
flub	flank	friar, fryer
flake	flunk	fresh
flock	flask	freeze
fluke	flaunt	froze
flick	flax	phrase
flag	flex	froth
flog	flinch	frank
fled	flint	France
flood	flirt	French
flat	fray	friend
fleet	free	frisk
flit	fro	fringe
flight	fry	front
float	frame	frost
flout	from	

The G Sound

The opposite of come is _____.	go
Going, going, _____.	gone
The opposite of bad is _____.	good
You go to church to worship _____.	God
The opposite of take is _____.	give
The opposite of guy is _____.	gal
The car needs a tank of _____.	gas
You have to take aim when you shoot a _____.	gun
A fish breathes through its _____.	gills
The house is haunted by a _____.	ghost
You have nothing to lose and everything to _____.	gain
Steady as she _____.	goes
It's not whether you win or lose, but how you play the _____.	game
The opposite of boy is _____.	girl
All that glitters is not _____.	gold
What's good for the goose is good for the _____.	gander

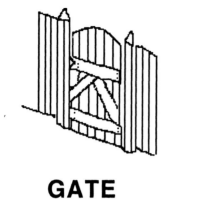
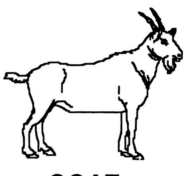
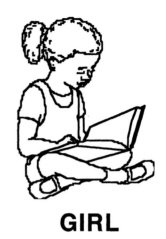

GATE   **GOAT**   **GIRL**

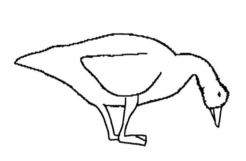
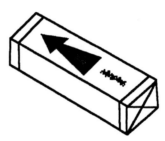
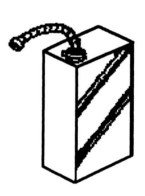

GOOSE   **GUM**   **GAS**

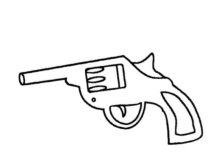
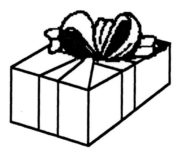
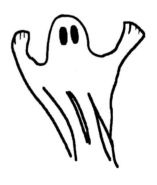

GUN   **GIFT**   **GHOST**

45

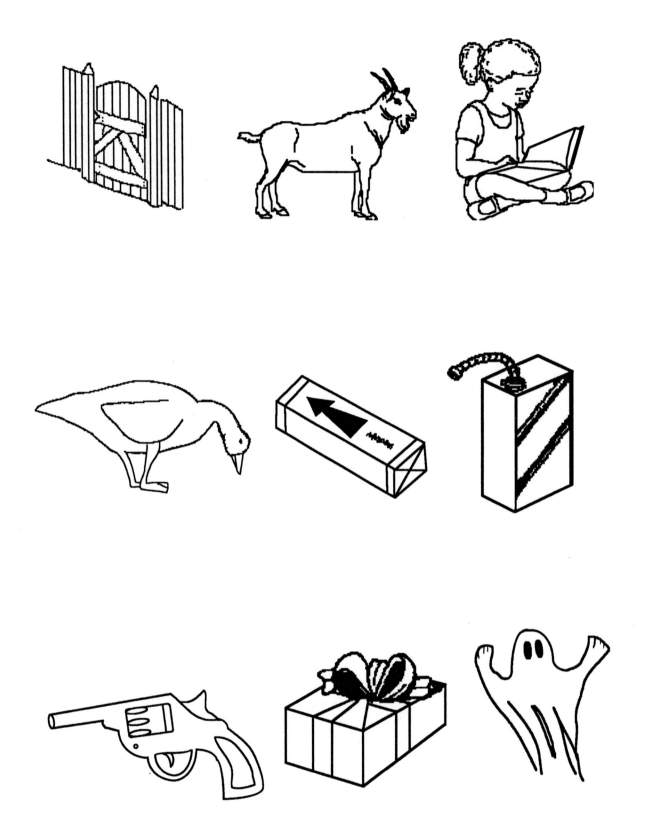

46

go	goat	gauze
goo	gout	guise, guys
gay	gut	gauge
gee	gang	gouge
guy	gaff	gave
gap	goof	give
gape	guff	ghost
game	gal	guest
gum	gale	gust
goon	gall	gasp
gown	ghoul	gift
gone	gill	gild, guild
gain	goal	gold
gun	guile	gimp
gab	gull	girl
gob	gar	girth
gawk	gear	gilt, guilt
gag	gas	gird
God, god	guess	gourd
guide	geese	guard
gaud	goose	golf
goad	gash	gulf
good	gosh	gorge
gate, gait	gush	gulch
get	gaze	gulp

go-go

good game

get gas

good guess

gag gift

gas gauge

golf game

give gifts

good girl

good gift

golf gear

gold gown

girl guide

guys and gals

get going

God given

go-getter

goose and gander

going good

gusty gale

golden girl

Golden Gate

guilty guy

garden gate

goody-goody

gobble goodies

Good guess, Gail.

good game of golf

Get going, Gus.

gotta get gas

going going gone

gaudy golden gown

Gus gave a gag gift.

Is checkers a book or a game?

Do you shoot a gun or a horn?

Is a saint bad or good?

Which is bigger, a frog or a goat?

Which is a fuel, gas or gum?

Which can fly, a goose or a goat?

Is a spook a ghost or a pet?

Which is more expensive, gold or lead?

Is it more blessed to give or receive?

Is a present a tax or a gift?

Does a fence need a door or a gate?

Is your best friend a guy or a gal?

Do you chew water or gum?

Which is bigger, a pond or the Gulf?

Is a wind a gale or a tide?

Do fish have gills or feet?

Is a mistake a goof or correct?

Is a wedding dress a tux or a gown?

Which can fly, a gull or a girl?

Is your sister a girl or a boy?

Which one is a sport, golf or chess?

When you push the gas pedal, does the car stop or go?

In soccer do you score a basket or a goal?

glee	grey, gray	grief
glow	grape	Grail
glue	grip	grill
glop	gripe	growl
gleam	grope	gruel
gloom	group	grace
glum	gram	grass
glean	grim	grease
glen	grime	gross
globe	groom	grouch
glib	grain	grave
glob	green	grieve
glad	grin	groove
glade	groan, grown	grove
glide	groin	growth
gloat	grab	grand
glut	grub	grind
glass	Greek	ground
gloss	grade	grant
glare	greed	grunt
glaze	grid	grasp
glove	greet	graft
gland	grate, great	grange
glance	grit	grump
glitch	graph	grudge
grow		

The H Sound

The opposite of low is _____.	high
Jack and Jill went up the _____.	hill
The opposite of cold is _____.	hot
You need to comb your _____.	hair
A group of cows is called a _____.	herd
People walk; rabbits _____.	hop
I live in a two-story _____.	house
Be it ever so humble; there's no place like _____.	home
The fingers and the palm are parts of the _____.	hand
The opposite of soft is _____.	hard
The opposite of love is _____.	hate
The opposite of heaven is _____.	hell
Little Boy Blue come blow your _____.	horn
You wear a hat on your _____.	head
Don't put your cart before the _____.	horse
One hundred percent is whole; fifty percent is _____.	half
When a person is deaf, he can't _____.	hear
You hit the nail on the _____.	head
Keep the news under your _____.	hat
Make yourself at _____.	home
Strike while the iron is _____.	hot
Blood is pumped by the _____.	heart
The opposite of sad is _____.	happy
He has a great sense of _____.	humor
The opposite of light is _____.	heavy

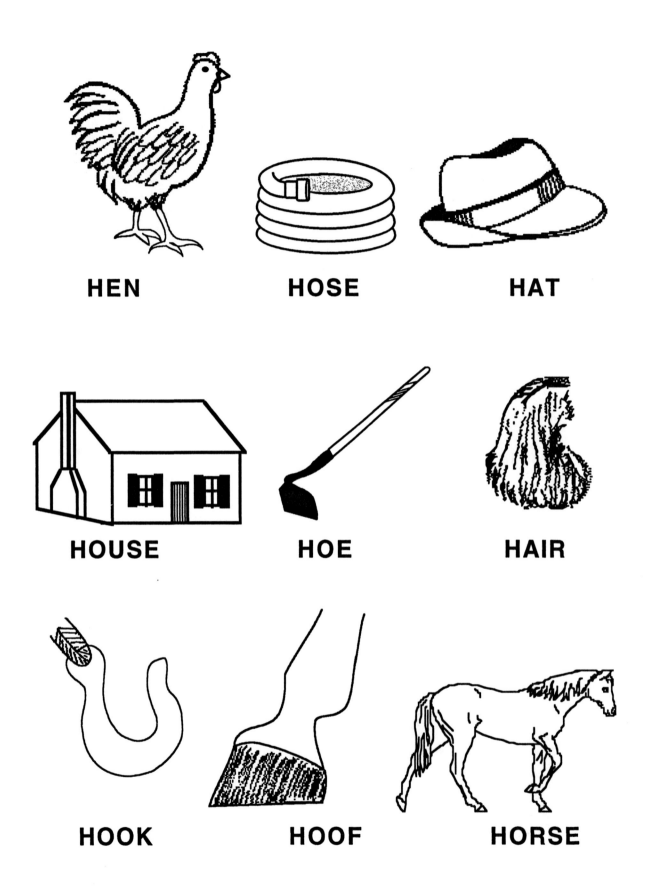

HEN HOSE HAT

HOUSE HOE HAIR

HOOK HOOF HORSE

52

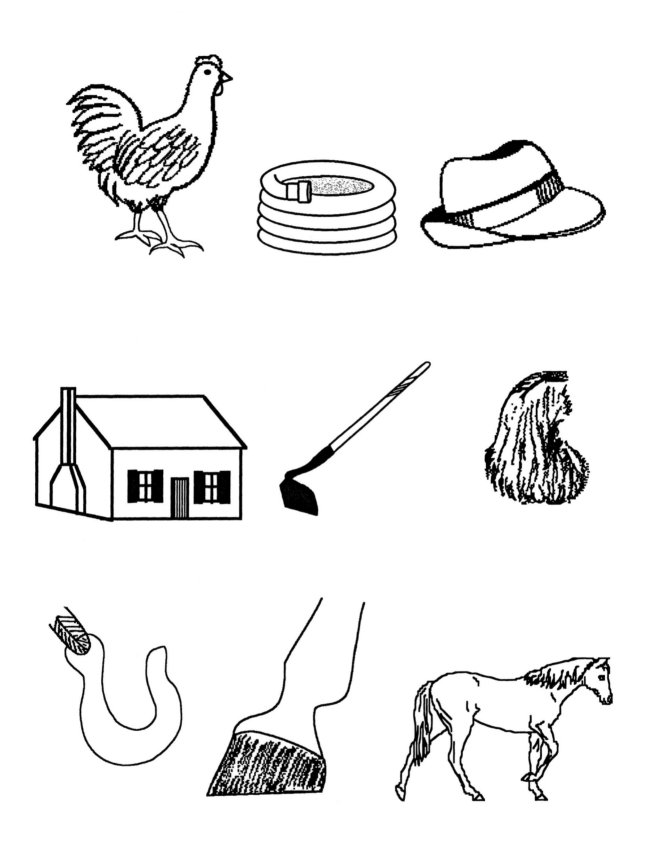

ha	hick	hall, haul
hay, hey	hike	heel, heal
he	hock	hell
hi, high	hook	hill
ho, hoe	hag	hull
how	hog	hole, whole
haw	head	hair, hare
hue, hew,	had	hire, higher
Hugh	heed	here, hear
heap	hid	house
hip	hide	hiss
hoop	hod	hooch
hop	hood	hash
hope	hat	hush
hype	hate	haze
ham	heat	hose
him, hymn	height	have
home	hit	heave
hum	hot	hove
hewn	hoot	hive
hen	hut	huge
hone	hung	heath
hub	hang	halt
hob	hoof	hilt
hack	huff	harp
hake	half	harm
hawk	hail	hark

hard	health
hoard	hearth
harsh	hedge
hatch	heist
hutch	host
hitch	hers
haunch	hex
haunt	hoax
hint	hold
halve	hoarse, horse
hand	horn
hind	hurl
hound	hurt
hank	hump
honk	hunt

heehaw	hardheaded
ho hum	hip huggers
high-hat	hard of hearing
hen house	hollyhock
ham hock	hurry home
heave ho	horror house
head home	hammerhead
high hopes	Hula-Hoop
hothouse	helping hand
hard hat	happy heart
household	happy home
hogshead	hobbyhorse
horsehair	hairy hound
hand-held	human hair
hitchhike	helpful hints
hold hands	heavyhearted
hired hand	harmful habit
huge herd	happy holidays
home health	hippity hop
half-and-half	He had help.
hard to hold	have high hopes
halfway house	her hired hand
halfhearted	hip, hip, hurrah
hotheaded	Hurry home, Hal.
hardhearted	He's house hunting.
highhanded	He is headed home.
house hunting	He's hardheaded.

He's hard of hearing.
Have a happy home.
Hardhearted Hannah
He is her hired hand.
He has to hurry home.
Hal has a heavy heart.

Do you live in a barn or a house?

Do you catch fish with a hook or a needle?

Does a rabbit hop or swim?

In August is it hot or cold?

Do pigs produce ham or steak?

Does a rabbit live in a hole or a nest?

Is fifty percent a half or a whole?

When you go bald, do you lose your hair or your teeth?

Is a group of cows a flock or a herd?

Is the blood pumped by the heart or the liver?

Is a rock hard or soft?

Which is smaller, a mountain or a hill?

Which is bigger, a goat or a horse?

Which is more expensive, a house or a TV?

Which is part of the foot, the heel or the palm?

Which is a farm animal, a hog or a bear?

Do horses eat hay or worms?

What do you do with your ears, hear or see?

Which is louder, a horn or a harp?

Are your eyes on your leg or your head?

Does a cow have a hoof or a shoe?

Do bees live in a cave or a hive?

Is a female chicken a rooster or a hen?

Is one hundred percent a half or a whole?

Is a mountain high or low?

Is the thumb part of the hand or the foot?

The J Sound

The boxer had a glass _____.   jaw

If you want to make money you get a good _____.   job

If you commit murder you will be put in _____.   jail

A well-known nursery rhyme is "Jack and _____."   Jill

For breakfast I ate cereal and drank a glass of orange _____.   juice

A deck of cards has 4 kings, 4 queens, and 4 _____.   jacks

The month after May is _____.   June

The month after June is _____.   July

I like peanut butter and _____.   jelly

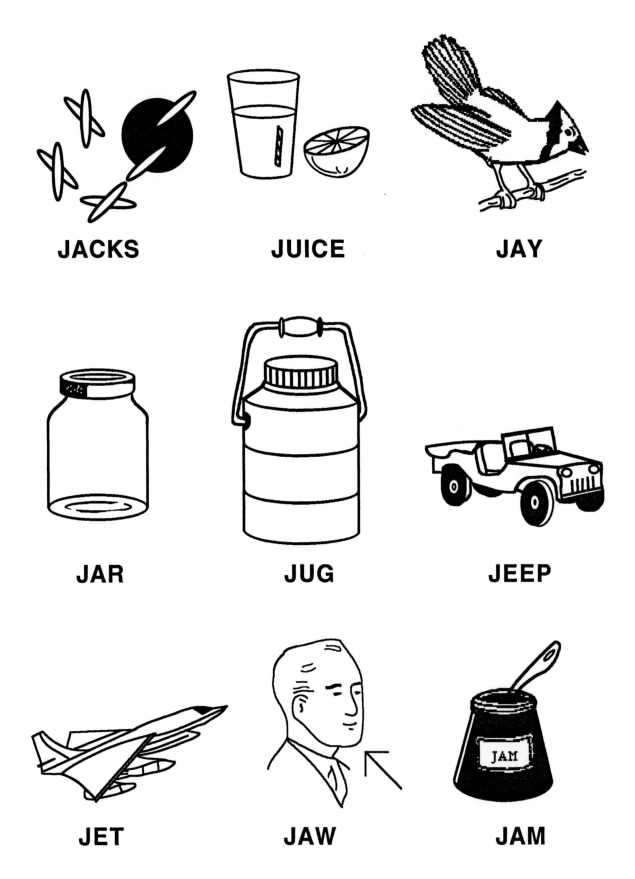

JACKS   **JUICE**   **JAY**

JAR   **JUG**   **JEEP**

JET   **JAW**   **JAM**

60

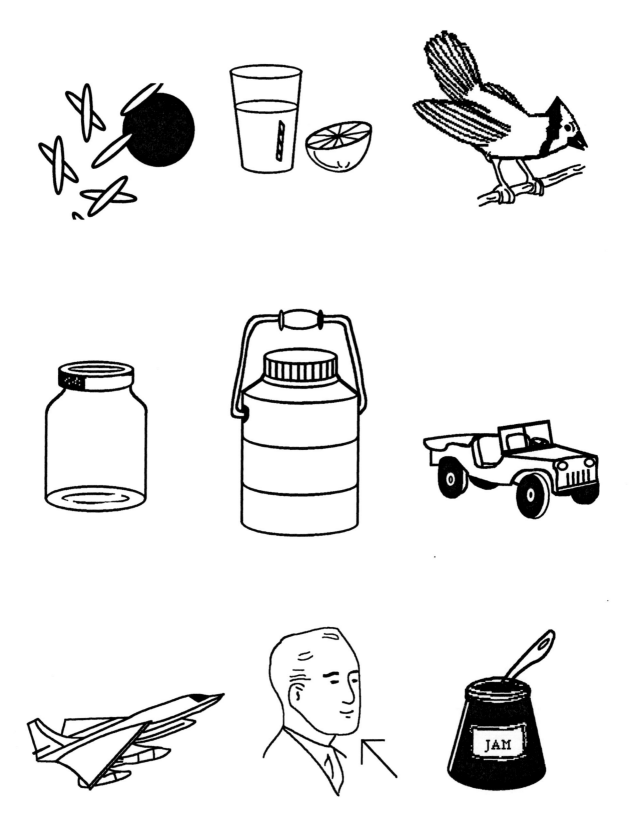

jay	jock	josh, Josh
jaw	joke	jazz
Joe	jag	judge
Jew	jig	jive
joy	jog	jaunt
jape	jug	gent
jeep	jade	joint
Jim, gym	Jude	jerk
gem	jet	germ
jam	jot	jest
gin	jut	joist
Jan	jute	joust
Jane	Jeff	just
Jean, gene	jail	jinx
John	jell, gel	jilt
join	Jill	jolt
June	Joel	jowl
jab	jar	July
jib	jeer	jump
jibe	jess, Jess	junk
job	juice	jury
jack, Jack		

jam jar

gin joint

jam and jelly

judge and jury

just joking

jumbo jet

jumping jack

ginger jar

genuine gem

Jo just joined.

John's gin joint

Jan and Jo jog.

Jill joked with Jan.

Jeff's just joking.

John just jammed the jar.

Which comes first, June or July?

Which is sweet, mustard or jam?

Which is a vehicle, a jeep or a chair?

Which is faster, a car or a jet?

Which is funny, a drama or a joke?

Which is hotter, October or July?

Which can you drink, juice or meat?

Which is part of the face, the jaw or the knee?

Which is bad luck, a jinx or a four-leaf clover?

Which is a dance, a jig or a song?

Which is a container, a rug or a jar?

Which is music, a poem or jazz?

Which drink is alcoholic, coke or gin?

Do runners jog or skip?

Which is a boy's name, Mary or John?

Which is a girl's name, Joe or Jane?

Which stone is green, jade or a ruby?

Does milk come in a jar or a jug?

Which one has twelve members, a trio or a jury?

The K Sound

How now brown _____.	cow
We keep our jewels under lock and _____.	key
If I'd known you were coming, I'd have baked a _____.	cake
It's your turn to shuffle the _____.	cards
You drink coffee from a _____.	cup
The bear lives in a dark _____.	cave
I like corn on the _____.	cob
He's rotten to the _____.	core
Go fly a _____.	kite
Put a feather in your _____.	cap
She's as nervous as a _____.	cat
Getting the stain out was a lost _____.	cause
We keep the canary in a bird _____.	cage
The water runs hot and _____.	cold
The opposite of go is _____.	come
Curiosity killed the _____.	cat
The opposite of hot is _____.	cold
The opposite of warm is _____.	cool
We locked the keys in the trunk of the _____.	car
The opposite of queen is _____.	king
A cow chews on her _____.	cud
Put these candles on the birthday _____.	cake
A baby goat is called a _____.	kid
Dots and dashes are used in Morse _____.	Code
That's a horse of a different _____.	color

65

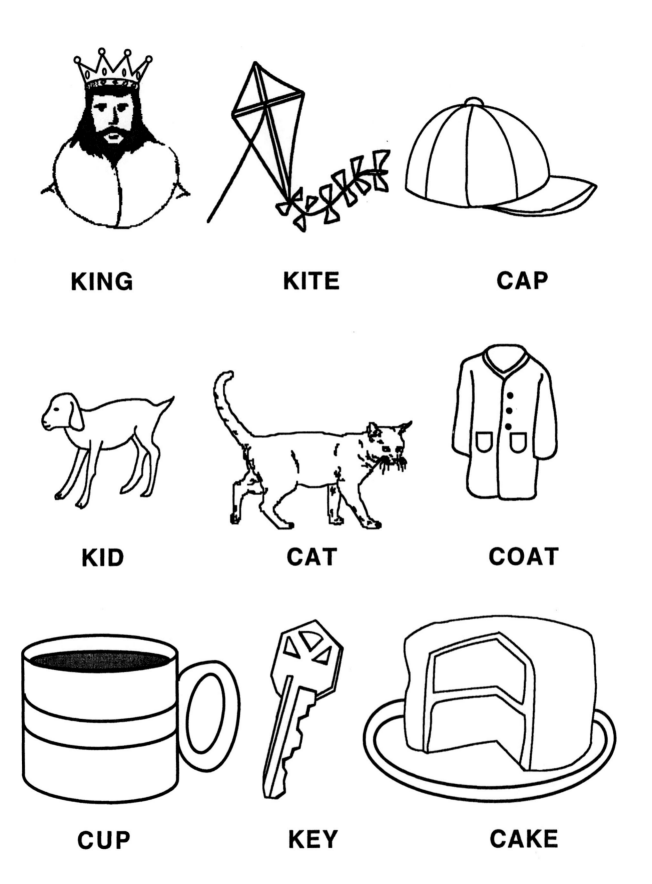

KING   **KITE**   **CAP**

KID   **CAT**   **COAT**

CUP   **KEY**   **CAKE**

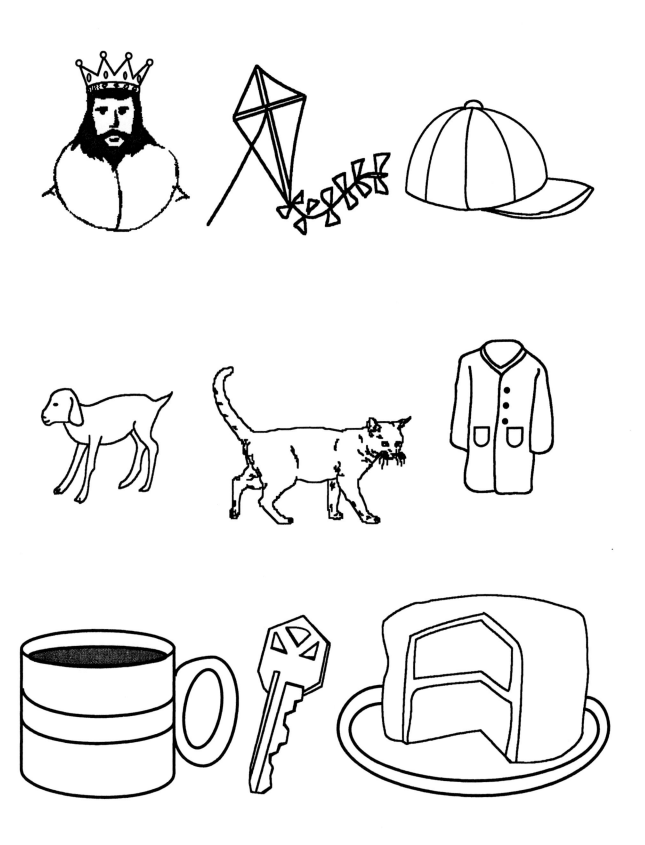

coo	cube	coal
cow	cake	coil
coy	cock	cool
cue	coke, Coke	cull
key	cook	kale
caw	kick	keel
cap	kook	kill
cape	cog	car
cop	keg	care
cope	cad	core
coup	cod	cure
cup	code	case
keep	could	cuss
cam	cud	kiss
came	kid	coach
comb	cat	cash
come	coat, cote	cause
can	cot	cage
cane	cut	cave
con, khan	cute	cove
coin	kit	kith
cone	kite	calk
coon	king	calm
keen	calf	camp
kin	cough	comp
cab	cuff	cant, can't
cob	call	count

card	cold
curd	conch
carp	cord
cart	colt
court	cult
curt	kilt
catch	conk
carve	kink
curve	cork
cast	curb
coast	curl
cairn	kelp
corn	kept
coarse, course	kerf
curse	kind
coax	

cold cash	coffee cup
King Kong	coffee cake
Coke can	cable car
copycat	candy cane
cute kid	carbon copy
cupcake	cozy kitten
corncob	Coca-Cola
cold cut	color coded
keep cool	cookie cutter
car key	cotton candy
catcall	cafe curtains
coal car	kissing cousin
cool cat	kitchen cabinet
catch cold	company car
cash-and-carry	calorie count
cut and curl	canary cage
kick a can	Can Carl cook?
keep coming	Carl can cook.
keep comfy	cold Coke can
cute kitten	Kate can catch.
cook cabbage	Kim's a cute kid.
count calories	Kick a Coke can.
cool and collected	cute kitty cat
calling card	keep cool and comfy
kitty cat	Kay carries cash.
carrot cake	Cars keep coming.
coffee can	Cook carrot cake.

keep a calorie count

Kay kept the car keys.

Carl can carry the case.

Carl can cook cabbage.

Kim cooked a carrot cake.

Does a canary live in a box or a cage?

Which is sweeter, bread or cake?

Which helps you walk, a cane or a skate?

Which goes on your head, a sock or a cap?

Do you drive a car or a wheel?

Which is feline, a dog or a cat?

Do bats live in holes or caves?

Who calls the plays, the coach or the water boy?

Which keeps you warm, a coat or a bikini?

Does corn grow on a pod or a cob?

Is a quarter a coin or a bill?

Does a chef paint or cook?

Do you like ice cream in a cup or a cone?

Does an apple have a core or a pit?

Do you drink coffee in a glass or cup?

Which is more pleasant, a slap or a kiss?

Which will fly, a brick or a kite?

Is October cool or hot?

Does beef come from a pig or a cow?

Which is a drink, a Coke or a cake?

Can you fly a rock or a kite?

Will scissors cut or paste?

Does a crow say caw or quack?

In spring is it cool or hot?

Does ice cream come in a cone or a jar?

claw	clung	croup
clay, Clay	cliff	cram
clue	clear	cream
clap	class	crime
clip	close	crumb
clop	clash	crane
claim	clause	croon
clam	cleave	crown
clan	clove	crab
clean	cloth	crib
clone	clamp	crack
clown	clomp	creek, creak
climb	clump	crick
club	clank	croak
clack	clink	crock
click	clasp	crook
cluck	clerk	crag
cloak	clinch	creed
clock	clench	crowd
clog	clutch	crude
clad	craw	crud
clod	crow	crate
cloud	crew	crawl
clot	cry	cruel
clout	crepe	crawl
cling	creep	creel
clang	crop	crass

cross

crease

crouch

crash

crush

craze

cruise

crave

craft

cramp

crimp

crank

crest

crust

crisp

crunch

crotch

crutch

crypt

The L Sound

The opposite of high is _____.   low

Let sleeping dogs _____.   lie

Murder is against the _____.   law

The opposite of early is _____.   late

A four-leaf clover is for good _____.   luck

The opposite of heavy is _____.   light

The opposite of cry is _____.   laugh

A chain is only as strong as its weakest _____.   link

The opposite of short is _____.   long

The opposite of quiet is _____.   loud

The opposite of hate is _____.   love

The opposite of right is _____.   left

At noontime we break for _____.   lunch

The opposite of win is _____.   lose

Last but not _____.   least

Jack Sprat could eat no fat; his wife could eat no _____.   lean

Keep a stiff upper _____.   lip

The opposite of first is _____.   last

Look before you _____.   leap

Live and let _____.   live

Mary had a little _____.   lamb

You'll have to read between the _____.   lines

Stop, look, and _____.   listen

Every dark cloud has a silver _____.   lining

The king of the jungle is the _____.   lion

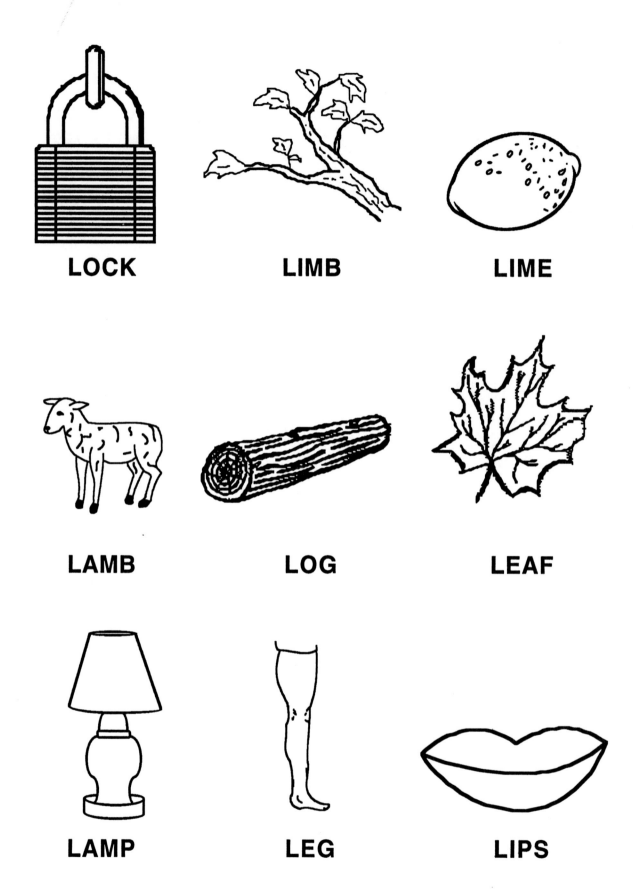

LOCK   **LIMB**   **LIME**

LAMB   **LOG**   **LEAF**

LAMP   **LEG**   **LIPS**

76

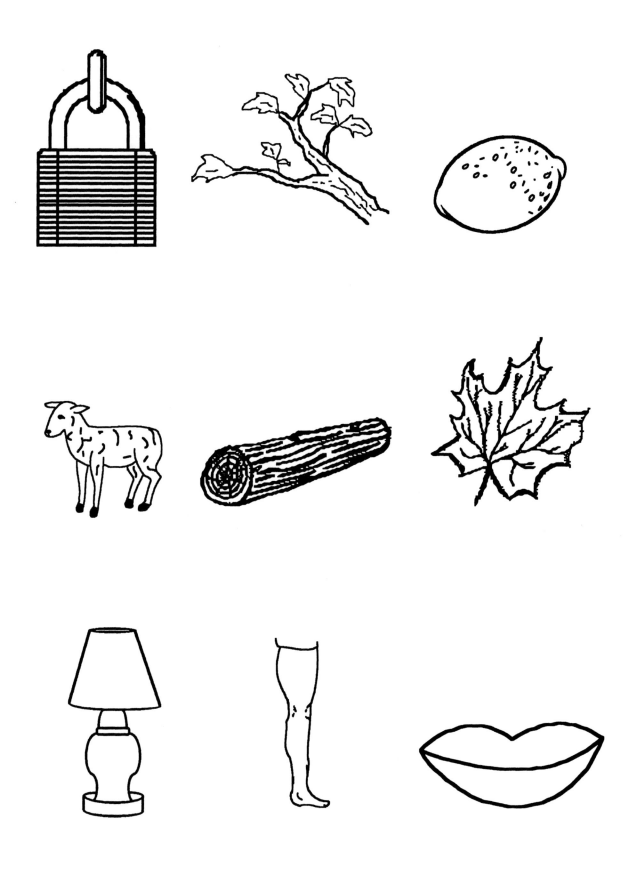

lay, lei	lobe	lot
lie, lye	lake	lout
low	lack	let
lee, Leigh	leak, leek	long
Lou, lieu	like	lung
law	look	laugh
lap	lick	life
lip	Luke	loaf
leap	lock	leaf
lop	luck	luff
lope	leg	loll
loop	lag	lull
lamb	log	lair
limb	lug	leer
lame	lad	lore
lime	laud	lure
loom	lead	lass
loam	load	lace
line	loud	less
lean, lien	lid	lice
loin	laid	loss
lone, loan	lewd	louse
loon	led, lead	lease
lawn	lied	loose
lain, lane	light	leach, leech
lab	late	loach
lob	loot, lute	lush

lash	lark
leash	lurk
laze	last
lose	lest
liege	list
live	least
leave	lost
love	lust
lath	latch
loathe	launch
lathe	lunch
lax	length
lox	learn
lamp	left
limp	lift
lump	loft
lank	lens
link	Lent, lent
lance	lint
land	lilt
lend	lisp
lapse	lodge
lard	lounge
lord	lurch
large	lynx

lie low	lift the lid
lifelike	light the lamp
lifeless	live lobster
lake loon	landlubber
lifeline	live lizard
light load	love letter
lame leg	landlady
limelight	light and lively
lifelong	look and listen
left lane	lick a lemon
left leg	life and liberty
let's live	lick a lollipop
long line	liver loaf
long life	Little League
last lap	a little late
last laugh	little lamb
lost lab	lemon lift
let's leave	lettuce leaf
large lake	lover's leap
leg lifts	lemon and lime
lick lips	lovely lady
light lunch	lucky lady
loose lips	leaping lizards
landlord	looping lasso
last leg	legal limit
landlocked	lily-livered
lots of luck	luminous lamp

late light lunch

Lou likes liver.

Let Lilly live.

Live a long life.

Let's look lively.

Let's live a little.

Lou loves Laura.

Lynn likes lemons.

little lost lamb

lovely large lake

Larry likes limes.

Lisa loves leopards.

legal liquor limit

Lynn is a lucky lady.

Let's live a long life.

Let's look a little lively.

Larry likes lemons and limes.

Which is sour, an apple or a lime?

Which is bigger, a lion or a cat?

Which is made up of water, a lake or a pasture?

Which is longer, your leg or your arm?

Is noon dark or light?

Is a drum loud or soft?

Does a tree have petals or leaves?

Which lives on water, a chicken or a loon?

Which needs a key, a hole or a lock?

Does bread come in a loaf or a deck?

Which is tamer, a tiger or a lamb?

Do you mow your floor or your lawn?

Which word means skinny, lean or fat?

Does a dog need a leash or a purse?

Which is better, love or hate?

Which is tatted, hose or lace?

Do banks make loans or bread?

Which is bigger, a stick or a log?

Which is bigger, a pond or a lake?

Which is straighter, a line or a circle?

Which is lighter, a leaf or a rock?

Is the Mississippi River long or short?

Do pencils have ink or lead?

Does a jar have a lid or a cap?

If you are renting, do you have a lease or a deed?

The M Sound

The month after April is _____.   May

One for you and two for _____.   me

A cow says _____.   moo

Out of sight, out of _____.   mind

We sang "Three Blind _____."   Mice

We sang "By the Light of the Silvery _____."   Moon

Don't cry over spilled _____.   milk

The opposite of woman is _____.   man

The sun comes out in the day; at night you see the _____.   moon

The opposite of less is _____.   more

The mailman delivers the _____.   mail

I'm as quiet as a _____.   mouse

Lamb, chicken, and beef are all kinds of _____.   meat

Lunch is the noontime _____.   meal

Here is one man. There are two _____.   men

There are 5,280 feet in a _____.   mile

I'll call Dad and _____.   Mom

Wipe your feet on the welcome _____.   mat

That man isn't nice, he is real _____.   mean

He's as stubborn as an old _____.   mule

They're so rich, they have a butler and a _____.   maid

The month after February is _____.   March

You can start a fire when you strike a _____.   match

Never look a gift horse in the _____.   mouth

Give him an inch and he'll take a _____.   mile

A rolling stone gathers no _____.   moss

When God made him he broke the _____.   mold

If you leave your ice cream in the sun, it is going to _____.   melt

I don't get paid until the end of the _____.   month

Don't spend all your _____.   money

You have a father and a _____.   mother

You get a job to make a lot of _____.   money

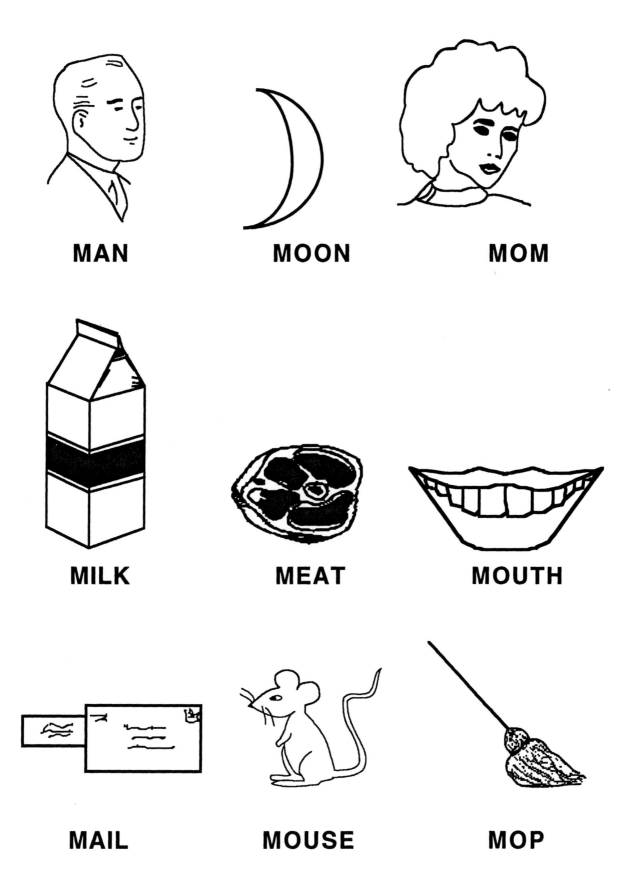

MAN   **MOON**   **MOM**

MILK   **MEAT**   **MOUTH**

MAIL   **MOUSE**   **MOP**

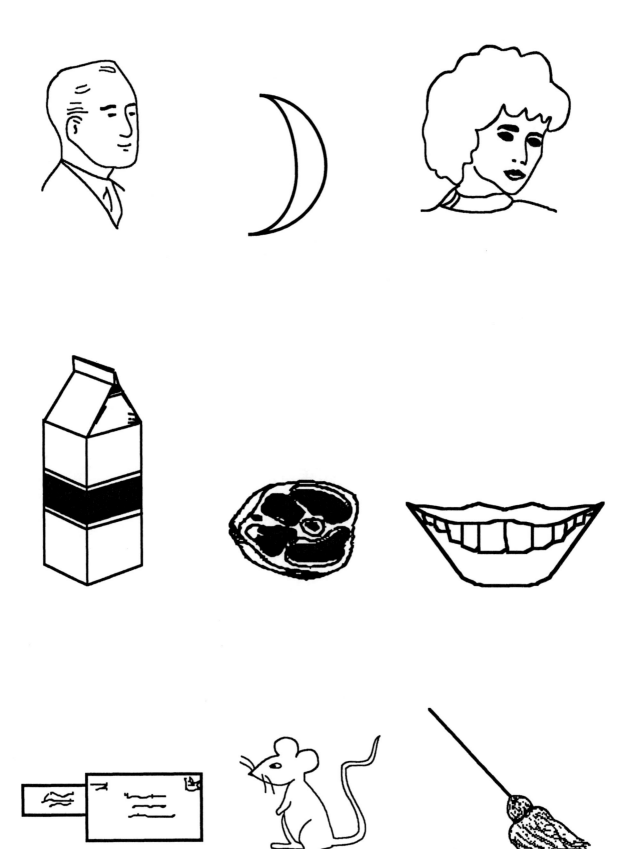

ma	mad	more
may, Mae	mod	mar
me	mood	mare
mow	mud	mire
moo	made, maid	moor
mew	mode	mere
maw	mead	mice
mope	mid	mass
map	mat	miss
mop	mate	mouse
ma'am	moat	mess
mom	mitt	muss
mum	might, mite	moose
mime	mutt	mace
main, mane	meat, meet	moss
men	met	mooch
mine	mute	much
moon	moot	mush
mean	miff	mash
man	mail, male	mesh
moan, mown	mall, maul	maze, maize
mob	mile	muse
mike, Mike	meal	move
make	mill	mauve
muck	mole	math
mock	mull	moth
mug	mule	myth

mouth	mend
malt	mind
melt	merge
molt	mild
march	mold
mark	mix
murk	milk
mart	mince
Mars	mint
marsh	meant
mask	mount
musk	mink
mast	monk
mist	morgue
most	morn, mourn
moist	month
must	mulch
match	munch

my mom	mile marker
my mail	mild-mannered
my meat	marshmallow
madman	make millions
mean man	make a mistake
mailman	mass media
man-made	malted milk
my mouth	many more
my milk	marry me
milkman	motorman
milkmaid	moldy meat
more milk	Minnie Mouse
mainmast	Mickey Mouse
main meal	malted milk
marksman	music man
mush mouth	married man
masked man	motor mouth
make a mess	mealy mouth
make merry	minuteman
matchmaker	middleman
my money	mastermind
make money	money-maker
more money	Monday morning

many more men
my main meal
make more meat
Mary made a mess.
make me a match
meet my mother
man-made motor
my mom's mother
much more money
make more money
mild-mannered man
Monday morning mail
Mike makes more money.
Meet my mom's mother.
My mom made a mistake.
My mom is making a mess.
Most mothers make the meals.
My mother makes muffins.
On Monday morning mail the message.

Which comes first, May or August?

Which do you put on cereal, milk or beer?

Which is older, a boy or a man?

Which is smaller, a bear or a mouse?

Which appears at night, the sun or the moon?

Which is female, your mother or your father?

Do you think with your foot or your mind?

Do you talk with your mouth or your leg?

Which is longer, a second or a minute?

Do you clean the floor with a mop or mud?

Which comes first, March or June?

Does the mailman deliver the mail or milk?

Does a cow moo or quack?

Is a boy a female or male?

Which is bigger, a dog or a mule?

Which is a planet, Mars or Alabama?

Which goes on the floor, a mat or a picture?

Is bacon a meat or a fruit?

Which is longer, a yard or a mile?

Which starts a fire, a witch or a match?

Which sounds better, music or noise?

Which is a boy's name, Mike or Betty?

Which is a girl's name, Mae or Bill?

Does the milkman deliver the milk or the mail?

Which is shorter, a year or a month?

Which lives under the ground, a mole or a mule?

The N Sound

The opposite of yes is _____.	no
The joint between the thigh and the calf is the _____.	knee
Out with the old, in with the _____.	new
I don't want to wait; I want it right _____.	now
Tie the rope in a square _____.	knot
A hammer is used to pound _____.	nails
You wear a tie around your _____.	neck
The opposite of far is _____.	near
You smell with your _____.	nose
You cut your meat with a _____.	knife
They are as different as day and _____.	night
The opposite of messy is _____.	neat
The opposite of nephew is _____.	niece
The number after eight is _____.	nine
Another name for 12 PM is high _____.	noon
The opposite of south is _____.	north
Pecans, walnuts, and almonds are all kinds of _____.	nuts
Dan Rather commentates the 6 o'clock _____.	news
A stitch in time saves _____.	nine
Thunder makes a loud _____.	noise
The opposite of all is _____.	none
Better late than _____.	never
The opposite of wide is _____.	narrow
You sew with a thread and a _____.	needle
Another name for five cents is a _____.	nickel

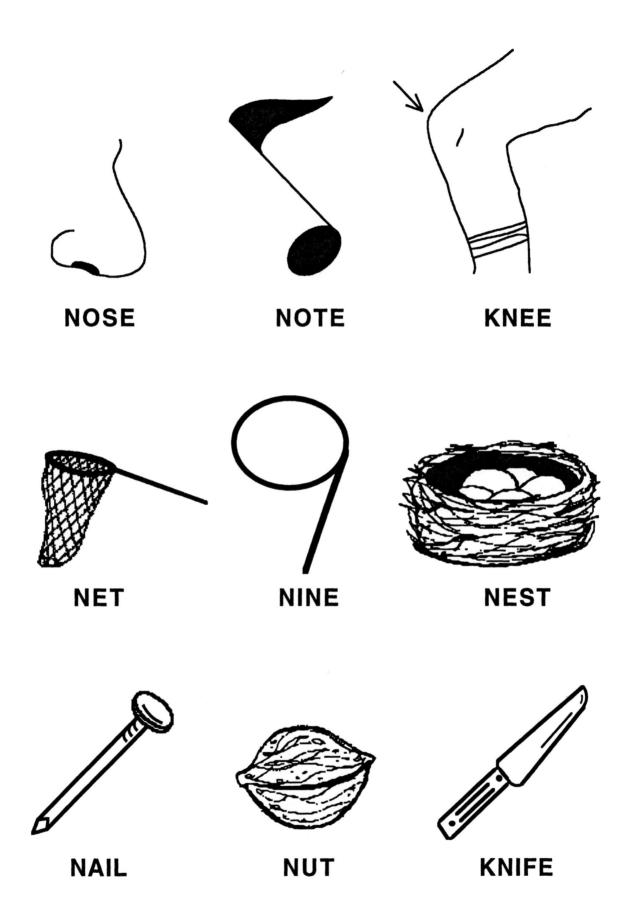

NOSE

NOTE

KNEE

NET

NINE

NEST

NAIL

NUT

KNIFE

93

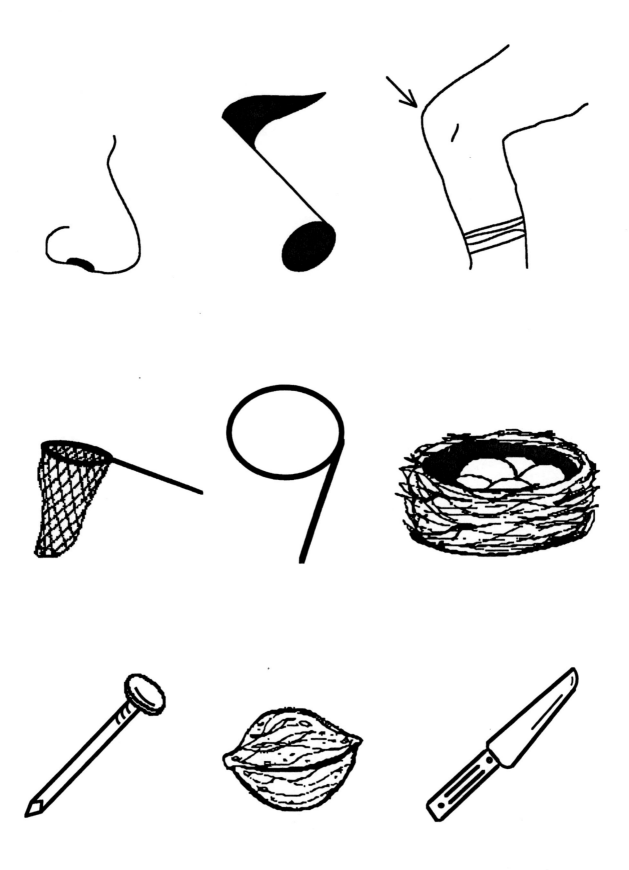

knee	nook	kneel
neigh	knock	null
gnaw	knack	nor
nigh	nag	near
no, know	need, knead	niece
new, knew	nod	nice
now	node	noose
nap	nude	gnash
neap	gnat	news
nip	not, knot	nose
name	neat	noise
numb	net	knave
gnome	night, knight	gnarl
noun	knit	nerve
none, nun	note	nest
noon	newt	next
nine	naught	notch
known	nut	norm
nab	knife	north
knob	nail	nurse
neck	nil	nymph
nick		

no name
new net
no news
nice nun
not now
new knife
nice night
nine notes
knock-kneed
nice niece
numb knee
knickknack
nickname
noble nurse
ninety-nine
naughty nephew
noisy neighbors
Not now, Nan.
nine new knives
no new news
nine neat nuns
Nick knew nothing.
ninety-nine knots
Nick noticed the nice note.
Nan bought nine new knives.

Does a necklace go around your waist or your neck?

Which is dark, night or day?

Which will bend, your thigh or your knee?

Do you smell with your ear or your nose?

Which is female, a niece or a nephew?

Which is 12 PM, noon or sunrise?

Which is Catholic, a rabbi or a nun?

Do you cut with a spoon or a knife?

Which number comes after eight, nine or ten?

Which is louder, a whisper or a noise?

Which has a sharp point, a nickel or a nail?

Is Maine in the north or the south?

Is a pecan a meat or a nut?

Do you catch fish in a net or a bucket?

Does the moon appear in the day or the night?

Which is worth five cents, a dime or a nickel?

Do you use yarn to tat or to knit?

Does a door have a receiver or a knob?

Is the word "uncle" a noun or a verb?

Is _(name)_ your name or your address?

Does a bird build a house or a nest?

Is a short rest a nap or a cap?

Does a horse neigh or bark?

Who works in a hospital, a nurse or a banker?

The P Sound

You have a ma and a _____.	pa
I baked an apple _____.	pie
At church I sit on the front _____.	pew
I like corn bread and black-eyed _____.	peas
Bacon comes from a _____.	pig
You cook eggs in a _____.	pan
Put on your shirt and _____.	pants
You write with a _____.	pen
The opposite of war is _____.	peace
Before you eat a banana, you take off the _____.	peel
Let's smoke the peace _____.	pipe
You push and I will _____.	pull
Boys wear blue; girls wear _____.	pink
A man carries a wallet; a woman carries a _____.	purse
The opposite of rich is _____.	poor
I cook soup in a _____.	pot
We had a picnic in the _____.	park
You stuck me with a _____.	pin
I'm as pleased as _____.	punch
Santa Claus lives at the North _____.	Pole
My grandfather smokes a _____.	pipe
All the bills have been _____.	paid
The opposite of tan is _____.	pale
I'm tickled _____.	pink
They are like two peas in a _____.	pod

98

This house needs a new coat of _____.   paint

You write on _____.   paper

Pass the salt and _____.   pepper

Ten cents is a dime; one cent is a _____.   penny

We are going to give a surprise birthday _____.   party

The thief was caught by the _____.   police

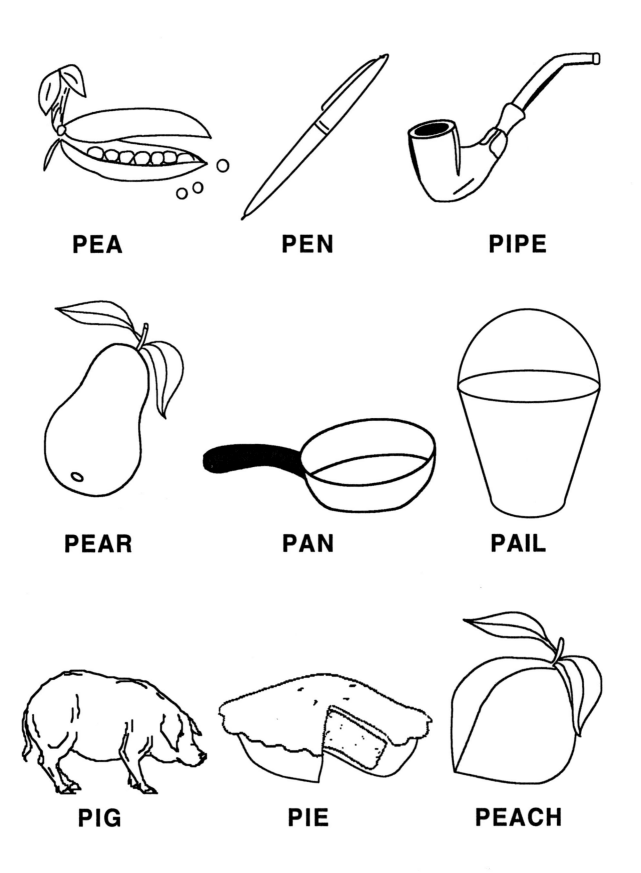

PEA　　　**PEN**　　　**PIPE**

PEAR　　　**PAN**　　　**PAIL**

PIG　　　**PIE**　　　**PEACH**

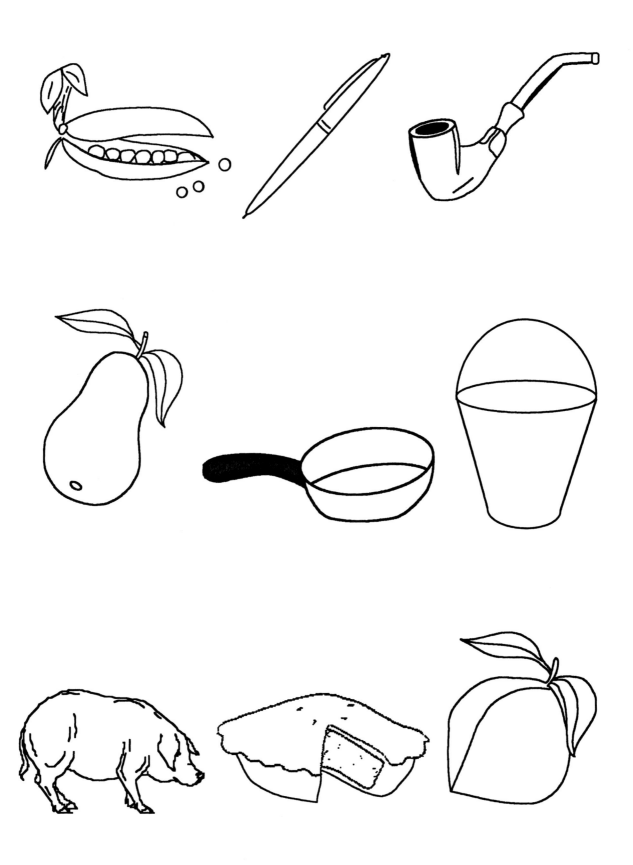

101

pay	pack	pile
pa	peek, peak	pill
pea	peck	pool
pie	pike	poll, pole
pooh	pick	pull
pew	poke	par
paw	peg, Peg	pair, pare, pear
pow	pug	peer, pier
pop	pig	pure
poop	paid	pour, pore
pep	pad	poor
Pope	pied	pace
peep	pod	pass
pup	pat, Pat	peace, piece
pip	pet	peach
pipe	peat, Pete	poach
Pam	pit	posh
pain	pot	push
pan	pout	pose
pawn	put	poise
pen	putt	pause
pin	ping	page
pine	puff	pave
pun	pal	peeve
pone	pail, pale	path
pub	pall, Paul	palm
pock	peel, peal	pearl

pant	post
paint	pact
pent	pelt
point	pence
punt	pink
patch	punk
pitch	pinch
park	punch
pork	pond
parse	pound
purse	pox
part	pulp
port	pulse
past	pump
paste	purge
pest	

pea pod

pigpen

ping-pong

potpie

pinpoint

pep pill

peach pie

peace pipe

pet peeve

postpone

passport

pitch pipe

pink paint

push and pull

pick a peach

piece of pie

pots and pans

pound of pork

pill popper

Pied Piper

pink panther

pour pepper

pickpocket

pinch pennies

pen and paper

pen and pencil

pay for pizza

paint a picture

peel a potato

Peter Pan

parcel post

perfect pair

pastel paint

public park

parrot perch

pinto pony

polo pony

public person

penny pincher

purple paper

pitter-patter

picture perfect

parallel park

pink pep pill

pork potpie

pay for pots and pans

ping-pong paddle

Pete's pet pony

postponed party

piece of pecan pie

pink and purple pants

push piano pedals

pick peaches and pears

Peter pays Paul.

Paul pushed and Pat pulled.

Pop pickled pears and peaches.

Pat poked Paul with a pin point.

Paul picked pecans for a pie.

Paul printed the purple paper.

Pat picked pastel paint.

Paul paid for a pound of pork.

Pay for the pink and purple pants.

Pop paid for the pots and pans.

Do you write with a pen or a match?

Do you smoke a pie or a pipe?

Which is a color, pink or paint?

Which is sharper, a pin or a finger?

Do you cook in a pot or a vase?

Which is worth one cent, a dime or a penny?

Which is a seasoning, pepper or meat?

Which is a boy's name, Peggy or Pete?

Does bacon come from a pig or a lamb?

Do you fry in a sink or a pan?

Does a banana have a peel or a core?

Which is clothing, a ring or pants?

Do women keep their money in a box or a purse?

Which is softer, a pillow or a wall?

Which do you drink, paint or punch?

Is what happened yesterday in the past or the future?

Which is bigger, a pony or a cat?

Which is a fruit, a pear or a potato?

Which is shorter, a poem or a novel?

Which has a zipper, socks or pants?

Which is a vegetable, peas or a peach?

Which can you erase, a pen or a pencil?

Which is bigger, a pint or a peck?

Which is a meat, beans or pork?

Do you swim in a pool or a tub?

Is a baby dog called a pup or a calf?

ply	place	prick
ploy	plush	proud
plow	please	prude
plea	plank	pride
play	plunk	prod
plum, plumb	plant	prong
plume	pledge	proof
plan	plump	prowl
plane, plain	plunge	press
plaque	pro	price
pluck	prow	preach
plug	pray, prey	praise, prays
plead	pry	prize, pries
pled	prop	prose
plod	prep	prove
plaid	prim	prance
plait	prime	prince
pleat	prawn	prank
plate	prune	primp
plight	prone	print
plot	preen	priest
plus	probe	

The R Sound

The opposite of cooked is _____.   raw

Two wrongs don't make a _____.   right

I smell a dirty _____.   rat

God formed Eve from Adam's _____.   rib

The opposite of smooth is _____.   rough

It is so cloudy, it will probably _____.   rain

The opposite of right is _____.   wrong

When she got engaged, she got an engagement _____.   ring

A block is square; a circle is _____.   round

The opposite of poor is _____.   rich

The opposite of walk is _____.   run

Oh, give me a home where the buffalo _____.   roam

My love is like a red, red _____.   rose

This bed is as hard as a _____.   rock

I'm as snug as a bug in a _____.   rug

I'm at the end of my _____.   rope

Let's go out and paint the town _____.   red

He'd complain if you hung him with a new _____.   rope

As you sow; so shall ye _____.   reap

Home, home on the _____.   range

Follow the yellow brick _____.   road

In school you learn to read and _____.   write

She's as nervous as a cat on a hot tin _____.   roof

My son listens to rock and roll music on the _____.   radio

I hear the telephone _____.   ringing

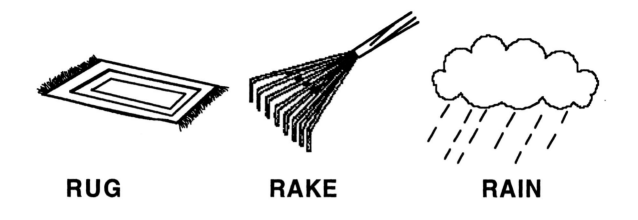

RUG **RAKE** **RAIN**

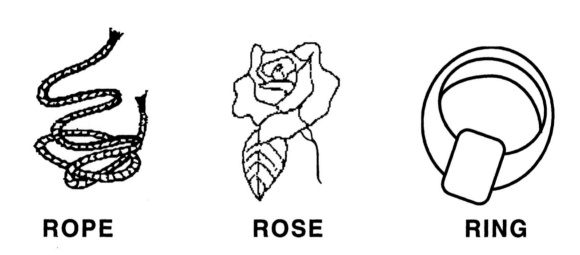

ROPE **ROSE** **RING**

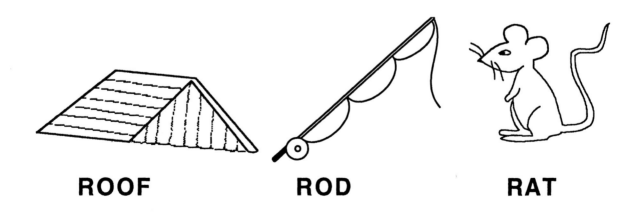

ROOF **ROD** **RAT**

109

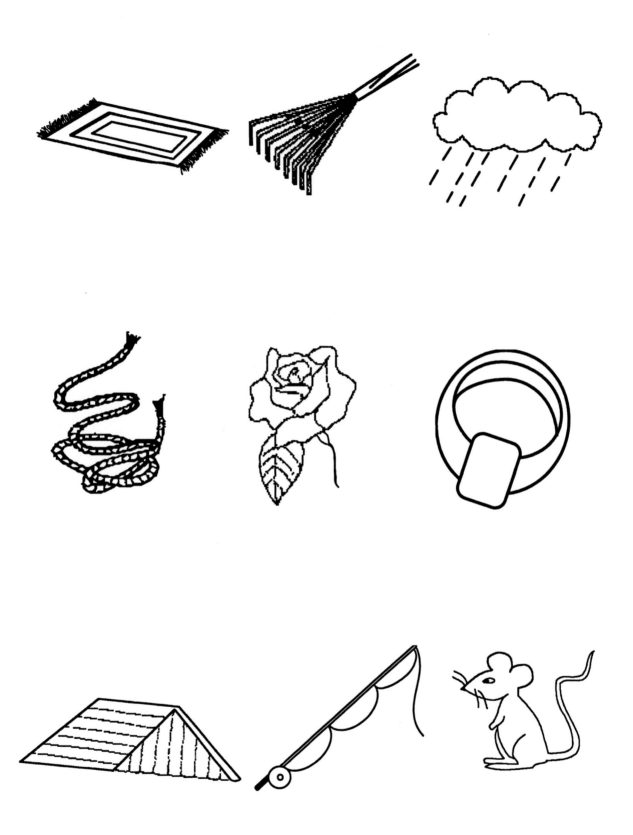

110

raw	robe	rote
ray	rub	ring, wring
rah	rack, wrack	rang
row, roe	rake	rung, wrung
rye	wreck, reck	wrong
roux, rue	reek, wreak	reef
rap, wrap	rick, Rick	rife
rape	rock	roof
reap	rook	rough, ruff
rep	rag	rail
rip	rogue	reel
ripe	rig	rule
rope	rug	rile
ram	raid	rill
ream	read, reed	role, roll
rim	red, read	roar
rum	ride	rear
roam	rid	rare
room	rude	rice
rhyme	road, rode	race
ran	rod	reach
rain, reign, rein	rat	rich
ruin	rate	roach
run	route, rout	rash
roan	right, rite, write	rush
rib	root, route	raise
rob	rot	razz

rise	rent
rose, rows	rasp
rouse	rend
rage	rind
rouge	wrench
rave	wretch
reeve	rest, wrest
rove	rust
rive	wrist
wrath	roast
ramp	roost
romp	ridge
rump	rinse
range	risk
rank	round
rant	rust

rat race

red rose

rough ride

rickrack

rip roar

rough rock

wrong room

riffraff

railroad

restroom

rump roast

rock and roll

read and write

rod and reel

right as rain

run a race

wreck and ruin

rant and rave

rule the roost

road rally

wrong reason

round robin

red radish

raw radish

roadrunner

rough-and-ready

rags to riches

rhyme and reason

rubber raft

rural road

rented room

roller rink

rifle range

Romper Room

ruby ring

river rat

razor rash

really rotten

rebel rouser

roaring rocket

regal ruler

Reading Railroad

red rickrack

ruby red rose

Ray reads rhymes.

Rob raised the roof.

Ray raises rice.

rough rural road

red razor rash

run a rapid race

right and wrong reasons

reading, writing, and
    arithmetic

Which smells sweet, a rose or garlic?

With measles, do you get a rash or a tumor?

Which is bigger, a mouse or a rat?

Is a millionaire rich or poor?

Which is an insect, a crow or a roach?

Which is red, mascara or rouge?

Is a circle square or round?

Which is a tool, a ball or a rake?

Is a book to read or to paint?

Is a car to ride or to fly?

Which is heavier, a feather or a rock?

Which is on top, the roof or the floor?

Do you drive on the sidewalk or the road?

Will a bell ring or honk?

Does an orange have a rind or a core?

Does a king reign or serve?

Is a vacation for work or rest?

Are black diamonds common or rare?

Which is a grain, soup or rice?

Which is bigger, a ram or a rat?

Do you wash with a napkin or a rag?

Which is brighter, red or black?

Which is alcoholic, rum or coke?

Does a thief murder or rob?

Does a ball roll or slide?

Is a kitchen a room or a vehicle?

The S Sound

You reap what you _____.   sow

There are plenty of fish in the _____.   sea

You cut wood with a _____.   saw

The opposite of happy is _____.   sad

The opposite of hard is _____.   soft

The opposite of north is _____.   south

You put your shoes on after your _____.   socks

Lemons and limes taste _____.   sour

Let's all sing a _____.   song

A nickel is worth five _____.   cents

You go to the doctor when you feel _____.   sick

Put the dirty dishes in the kitchen _____.   sink

The man bought a new pin striped, three piece _____.   suit

Like father, like _____.   son

Wash your hands with this bar of _____.   soap

The opposite of buy is _____.   sell

The number after five is _____.   six

The number after six is _____.   seven

The opposite of winter is _____.   summer

The opposite of cloudy is _____.   sunny

For breakfast I had a bowl of _____.   cereal

He swallowed the story hook, line, and _____.   sinker

Spring, summer, fall, and winter are the four _____.   seasons

This coffeepot is sterling _____.   silver

The opposite of brother is _____.   sister

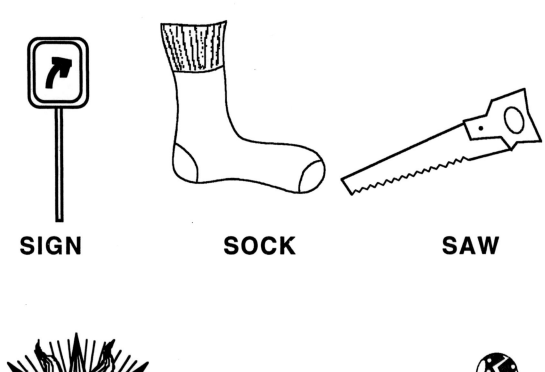

SIGN   **SOCK**   **SAW**

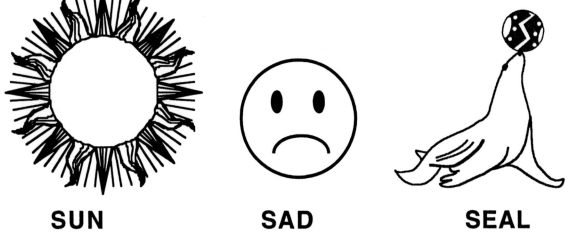

SUN   **SAD**   **SEAL**

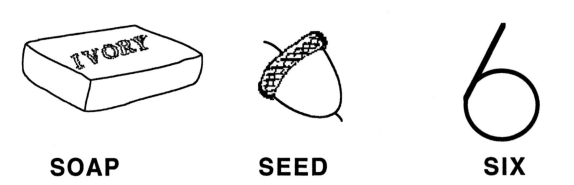

SOAP   **SEED**   **SIX**

116

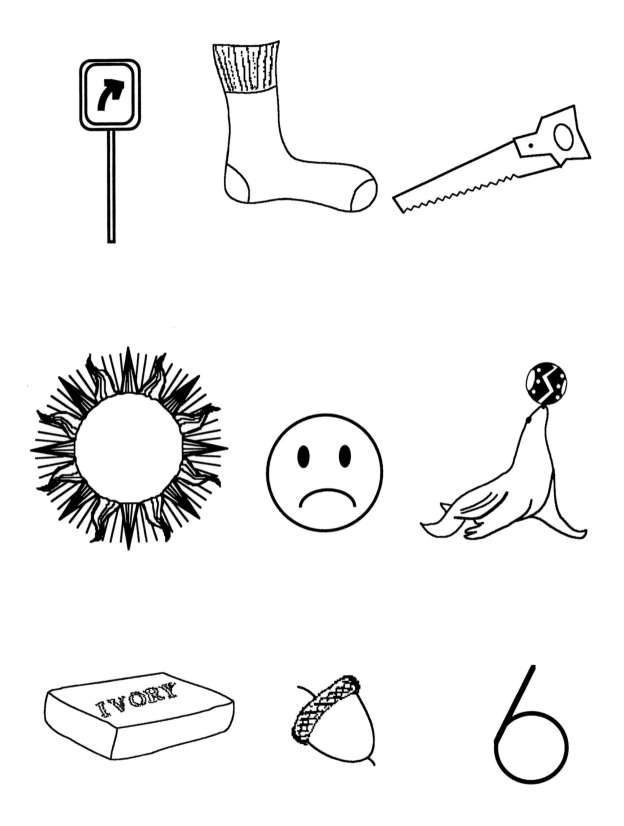

117

say	seek	soul, sole
see, sea	sake	sail, sale
sigh	sick	sear
so, sew, sow	sock	sir
sue, Sue	soak	sire
soy	sag	soar, sore
sow	sad	sour
saw	said	sass
soap	seed	sis
soup	side	sauce
sop	sod	such
sap	sat	sash
seep	sit	size
sip	seat	seize
sup	set	sage
seam, seem	sight, cite, site	siege
same	soot	save
some, sum	sought	sieve
Sam	suit	south
sane	sing	seethe
seen, scene	sang	soothe
soon	sung	saint
sign	song	salt
son, sun	safe	sand
sob	seal	send
sub	soil	sound
sack, sac	sell	sect

self

sex

six

socks

sent, scent

sense, cents

since

serve

silk

sink

sank

sunk

singe

soft

sword

sort

suds

surf

so sad

say so

so soon

seasick

soy sauce

sunset

seesaw

seaside

south side

sad song

sea surf

some soap

save cents

soak socks

soft sand

soapsuds

sixth sense

safe and sound

set of six

sightseer

some cider

sick sailor

self-service

sidesaddle

self-seeking

seersucker

sapsucker

sea serpent

six sisters

sunny side

sandy soil

somersault

seventh son

super sale

Caesar salad

semicircle

Simple Simon

civil service

salty celery

Social Security

sincere sympathy

six seesaws

so seasick

save six cents

sing a sad song

so safe and sound

Sam is safe and sound.

seasick sailor

some salty sauce

soft sandy soil

seersucker suit

super summer sale

sixty-six seals

seventy-seven songs

Sam has six sisters.
Sid sang a sad song.
Sandy saved sixty cents.
Sally said Sam said something.
Sam sat on the soft seat.
Some songs we sing are sad.

121

Which appears in the day, the sun or the moon?

Is a pair the same or different?

Is a lemon sweet or sour?

Is Florida in the north or the south?

Which goes on your foot, a sock or a glove?

If you are ill, do you feel sick or well?

Do you wash with soap or glue?

Does a tree have blood or sap?

Does a horse wear a cap or saddle?

Does a man wear a suit or a dress?

Is a penny a cent or a dollar?

When you cry, are you sad or happy?

Do you cut wood with a knife or a saw?

Is Mississippi in the north or south?

Is half a dozen four or six?

Are a needle and thread used to sew or to paint?

Should a boat sail or sink?

At night does the sun rise or set?

Are marshmallows soft or hard?

Is the Mediterranean a river or a sea?

Which number is larger, six or seven?

Is it hotter in the winter or summer?

Which one do you eat with a spoon, soup or steak?

Which one do you sing, a song or a story?

Which one can run under the water, a boat or a sub?

Which is a boy's name, Sue or Sam?

Does a bank keep the money in a safe or a jar?

skew	score	slum
ski	scour	slime
sky	scald	slain
scope	scold	slab
scoop	scalp	slob
skip	scamp	slack
scum	skimp	slake
skim	scarce	sleek
scan	scarf	slick
skein	scorch	slag
skin	scorn	slug
scab	Scotch	sled
skid	scowl	slide
scat	skirt	slat
scoot	skunk	slate
scout	slow	sleet
skate	slaw	slight
skeet	slay, sleigh	slit
skit	slew	slot
skiff	sly	slut
scoff	slap	sling
scale	sleep	slang
skill	slip	slough
skull	slope	slur
school	slop	slice
scar	slam	slouch
scare	slim	slash

123

slosh	smudge	snitch
slush	snow	snort
slave	snoop	spa
sleeve	snap	spay
sloth	snip	spew
slant	snipe	spy
slept	snob	span
slump	snub	spin
slink	snack	spine
slurp	snake	spawn
smack	sneak	spoon
smock	snag	spun
smoke	snug	speak
smog	snide	speck
smug	snit	spoke
smut	snout	spook
smite	snoot	spike
small	snuff	spade
smell	sniff	speed
smile	snail	sped
smear	sneer	spud
smooch	snare	spat
smash	snore	spit
smith, Smith	sneeze	spite
smooth	snooze	spot
smart	snarl	spout
smirk	snatch	spoof

spell	stem	still
spill	stain	stole
spoil	stone	stool
spool	stun	stair, stare
spar	stab	star
spare	stub	steer
spear	stack	stir
spore	stake, steak	store
space	stick	stash
spice	stuck	stage
speech	stock	stooge
spank	stag	stave
spunk	staid, stayed	stove
spark	stead	stalk
spent	stood	stamp
sponge	stud	stump
sport	stat	stance
spurn	state	stand
stay	stout	starch
stew	sting	stark
stow	staff	stork
sty	stiff	start
step	stuff	starve
steep	stale	staunch
stoop	stall	stern
stop	steal, steel	stilt
steam	style, stile	stink

125

stitch

storm

stunt

sway

swap

sweep

swipe

swoop

swim

swan

swine

swoon

swab

swag

sweet, suite

sweat

swat

swing

swung

swill

swell

swear

swore

Swiss

swish

suave

swamp

swank

swarm

swerve

swept

swift

swirl

switch

sworn

The Sh Sound

The opposite of he is _____.	she
He needs a haircut and a _____.	shave
Little Bo-Peep has lost her _____.	sheep
Make hay while the sun _____.	shines
The opposite of dull is _____.	sharp
After your socks, you put on your _____.	shoes
Halt, or I'll _____.	shoot
The opposite of tall is _____.	short
He works on the 3:00 to 11:00 work _____.	shift
The nurse gave him a penicillin _____.	shot
When he touched the plug, he got an electric _____.	shock
A snail lives in a _____.	shell
He is as white as a _____.	sheet
The opposite of open is _____.	shut
The opposite of whisper is _____.	shout
The opposite of deep is _____.	shallow

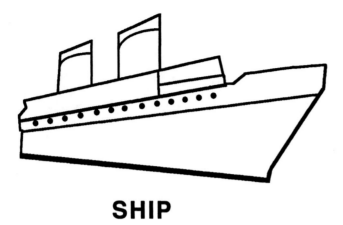

SHIP

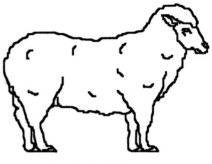

SHEEP

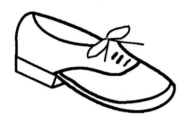

SHOE

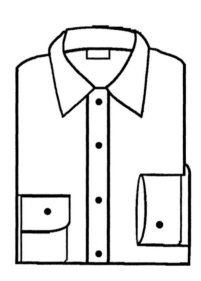

SHIRT

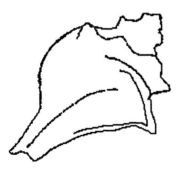

SHELL

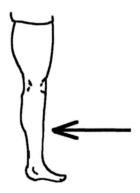

SHIN

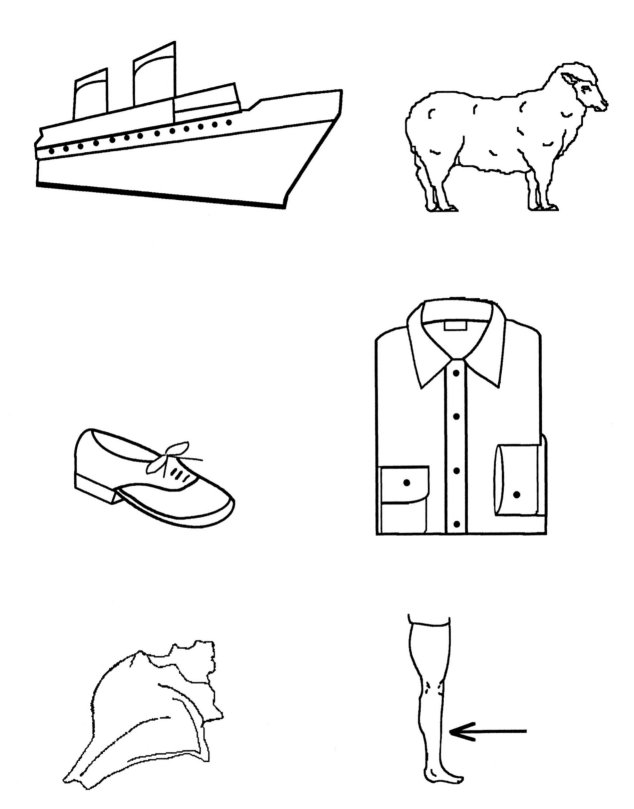

129

shay	shook	shire
she	shag	shirr
shoe, shoo	shad	shore
shah	shade	shush
show	shed	shave
shy	shod	shove
shape	should	sheave
sheep	sheet	sheath
ship	shoat	shaft
shop	shoot, chute	shift
sham	shot	shank
shame	shout	shard
shim	shut	shark
sheen	sheaf	shirk
shin	chef	sharp
shine	shale	shelf
shone, shown	shall	shelve
shun	shawl	shirt
shack	shell	short
shake, sheik	shill	shield
chic, sheik	shoal	shorn
shock	share	shunt
shuck	shear, sheer	

shoe shine

shell shock

sure shot

shoe shop

shipshape

she's short

shear sheep

sheep shank

shield shape

short show

ship to shore

shoot a shotgun

sharpshooter

shiny shoes

shabby shack

shiver and shake

shower and shave

shampoo and shave

shilly-shally

sugar shaker

She should share.

She should shop.

Shane shears sheep.

Shane's a sure shot.

She's short and shy.

Should she shower?

She should shower.

She shoots a shotgun.

shower, shampoo, and shave

She shears shaggy sheep.

Which is painful, a shot or a kiss?

Which produce wool, dogs or sheep?

Which goes on the bed first, the blanket or the sheet?

Which one floats, a ship or a car?

Which has sleeves, a shirt or a sock?

Does an oyster have a shell or a coat?

Do you use a razor to shave or to paint?

Do trees provide sun or shade?

Is the beach by the shore or the mountains?

Which is bigger, a guppy or a shark?

Is a midget tall or short?

Is a tack dull or sharp?

Does a coal mine have an attic or a shaft?

When you clean oysters, do you shuck or pluck?

Do you dig with a rake or a shovel?

When you take a bath, is the drain open or shut?

Will a gun shoot or sprinkle?

Is a lamb bold or shy?

Do you park your car in the kitchen or the shed?

Which is rock, shale or glass?

If you are cold, do you shake or sweat?

The T Sound

One plus one equals _____.	two
You can't eat your cake and have it _____.	too
The opposite of short is _____.	tall
The opposite of bottom is _____.	top
Before you get married you take a blood _____.	test
All I want for Christmas is my two front _____.	teeth
The number after nine is _____.	ten
Two thousand pounds equals one _____.	ton
Open your mouth and stick out your _____.	tongue
You take a bath in the bath_____.	tub
A clock is for telling _____.	time
The opposite of wild is _____.	tame
My car has a flat _____.	tire
The federal government collects an income _____.	tax
The opposite of give is _____.	take
This is a one horse _____.	town
Stick the bow on with Scotch _____.	tape
Only time will _____.	tell
The dog wagged his _____.	tail
The Dallas Cowboys is a football _____.	team
Marriage is a lot of give and _____.	take
My cousin lives in Dallas, _____.	Texas
When we were in Paris, we saw the Eiffel _____.	Tower
Another word for cab is _____.	taxi
Put all your cards on the _____.	table

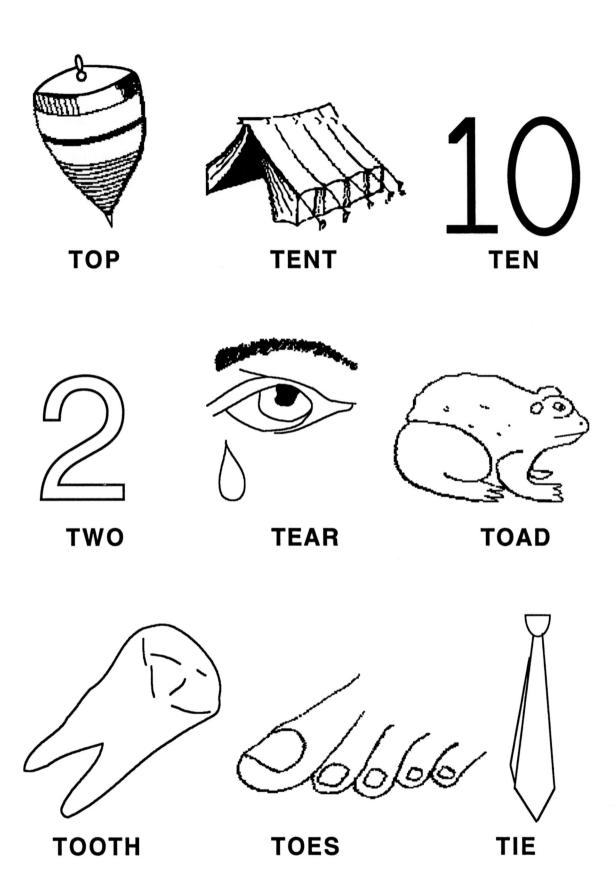

TOP

TENT

TEN

TWO

TEAR

TOAD

TOOTH

TOES

TIE

134

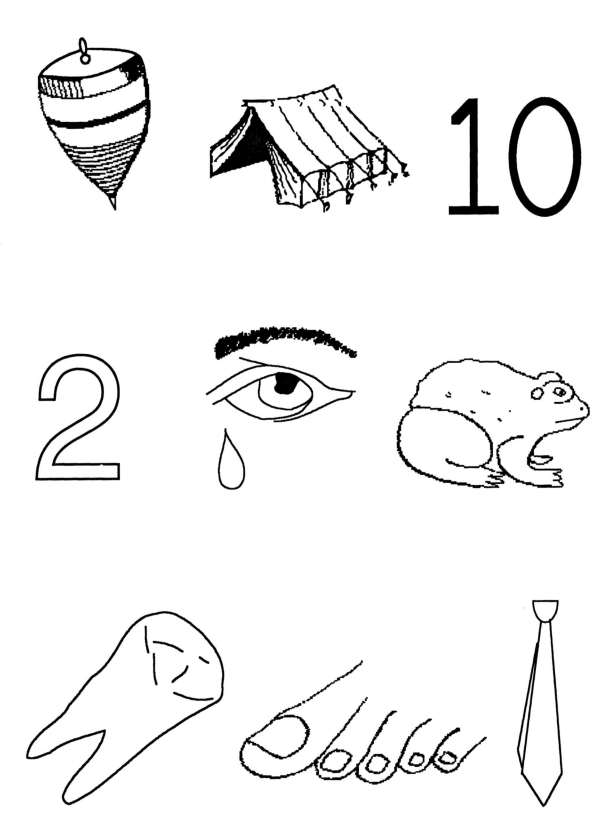

taw	tab	tell
to, too, two	tube	tile
tea, tee	tub	till
toy	tack	toil
tie, Thai	take	toll
toe, tow	tick, tic	tool
tap	took	tar
tape	tuck	tear
taupe	tag	tare, tear
tip	tog	tire
top	tug	tour
type	tide	toss
tam	toad	teach
tame	tot	touch
team	tote	tease
time, thyme	tat	tooth
tomb	taut, taught	teeth
tom, Tom	tight	talk
tan	tout	tamp
ten	toot	tank
tin	tong	tart
tine	tongue	tort
tone	tiff	task
ton	tough, tuff	tusk
town	tail, tale	taste
tune	tall	test
teen	teal	toast

taunt

tent

tint

tax

tux

term

tend

tense

turn, tern

tilt

told

torch

tuft

turf

tiptop

tiptoe

tom-tom

tea time

tie tack

toy tank

take two

tell time

tall teen

take time

tube top

tag team

ticktock

touch-tone

test tube

tilt-top

take turns

too tired

tongue-tied

taste test

toss and turn

turntable

too tiny

tame tiger

team teaching

two-timing

talk turkey

two tablets

timetable

ticker tape

tinker toy

tattletale

tinsel town

tiger tooth

table top

teeter-totter

table tennis

topsy-turvy

toilet tissue

temper tantrum

tied too tight

ten 'till two

two times two

take two tablets

tic-tac-toe

tip top team

two ton tank

too tired today

tilt-top table

tongue-tied tenor

tell Tiny Tim

touch-tone telephone

Take time to talk.

Tom took a taste test.

Teach me to tell time.

Tim is the tallest tenor.

Tell Tom to talk to Tess.

139

Which is smaller, a town or a city?

Which is larger, number ten or two?

Is a pet tame or wild?

Which is a sport, tennis or knitting?

Which is a part of the foot, a finger or a toe?

Do you chew with your teeth or your lips?

Does a clock tell the news or the time?

Do you bathe in a sink or a tub?

Which is younger, a teen or an adult?

Which is wilder, a dog or a tiger?

Which is sharper, a tack or a tie?

When you make lace, do you tat or tap?

Which do you wear around your neck, a tie or a belt?

Is a duet made up of one or two?

Is a giraffe short or tall?

Which has caffeine, tea or milk?

In the sun do you get a tan or pale?

Does toothpaste come in a jar or a tube?

Which is sticky, tape or foil?

Does a tutor teach or sing?

Do your hands touch or taste?

Does a clock rattle or tick?

Is a saw a tool or a dish?

Is a lemon sweet or tart?

Which is made of bread, juice or toast?

Does your tongue hear or taste?

true	trod	trump
trow	trot	trance
tray, trey	trait	trench
tree	treat	trend
try	trout	trunk
trap	trough	trust
trip	trail	trudge
tripe	trawl	twin
troop, troupe	trial	twine
tram	trill	twig
trim	troll	tweed
train	trace	twit
tribe	tress	tweet
track	truce	twang
trick	truss	twill
truck	trash	twice
trig	troth	twinge
trade	truth	twirl
tread	tract	twist
tried	tramp	

The Th Sounds

You have four fingers and a _____.	thumb
First, second, _____.	third
Don't give it a second _____.	thought
Every rose has its _____.	thorn
The opposite of thin is _____.	thick
The opposite of thick is _____.	thin
A penny for your _____.	thoughts
Rich man, poor man, beggar man, _____.	thief
You sew with a needle and _____.	thread
One, two, _____.	three

thigh	thou	three
thaw	thy	threw, through
thumb	though	throw
theme	the	throne, thrown
thin	thee	throb
thick	they	thread
thug	them	throat
thud	then	threat
thought	than	throng
thing	thine	thrill
thief	that	thrice
thieve	their, there	thrash
thank	this	thrush
think	these	thresh
third	those	thrive
thorn	thence	thrift
thatch		thrust
theft		
thump		

Which one is part of the hand, the eyes or the thumb?

On a hot day does ice freeze or thaw?

Which one breaks the law, a thief or a preacher?

Which one grows on a rose bush, a thorn or a cone?

Which one is a small number, twenty or three?

Is a string thick or thin?

Does the brain think or pump blood?

Is syrup thick or thin?

The V Sound

I'd like a room with a good _____.	view
The bride covered her face with a _____.	veil
We moved our furniture in a moving _____.	van
Put the flowers in a _____.	vase
Grapes grow on a _____.	vine
Blood is carried in arteries and _____.	veins
If you shout too loud you will get a hoarse _____.	voice
The check was null and _____.	void
When you turn 18 years old, you can register to _____.	vote
Banks keep the money locked in a _____.	vault
Baby beef is called _____.	veal
When you get married, you have to say wedding _____.	vows
A three-piece suit comes with a jacket, pants, and a _____.	vest
How green was my _____.	valley
Dracula is a well-known _____.	vampire
He has a lot of vim and _____.	vigor
Jonas Salk discovered the polio _____.	vaccine

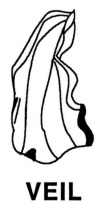

VEIL

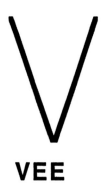

VEE

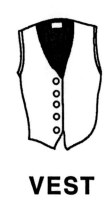

VEST

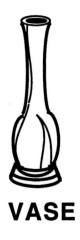

VASE

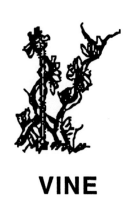

VINE

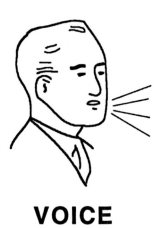

VOICE

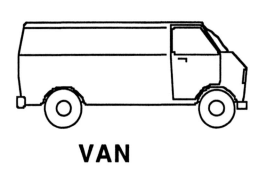

VAN

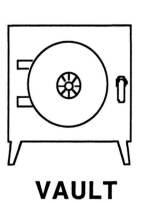

VAULT

146

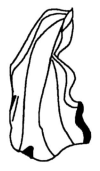
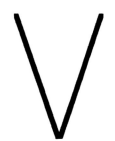
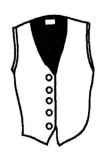

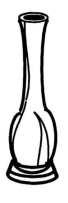
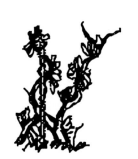
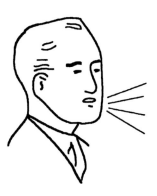

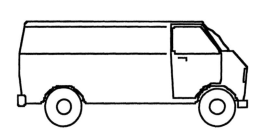
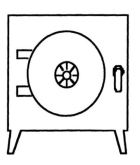

147

vie	vase
vow	vice, vise
view	voice
vim	vouch
van, Van	vamp
vain, vein, vane	vast
vine	vest
vague	vault
vogue	volt
void	valve
vat	vaunt
vet	vent
vote	vend
veal	verb
veil, vale	verge
vile	verse
veer	vex

vain vamp

vice versa

vast valley

vague victim

vim and vigor

violet vest

vibrant voice

very vicious

very verbose

vivid violets

virus vaccine

vicious vampire

vulgar Viking

veering vehicle

vicious and violent

valuable vase

varicose vein

violent varmint

venomous viper

very vain vamp

very valuable vase

Do grapes grow on a bush or a vine?

To elect someone to an office, do you vote or appoint?

Which is a vehicle, a basket or a van?

When you marry, do you make a wish or a vow?

Does a bride wear a helmet or a veil?

Do you speak with a voice or a whistle?

Does blood flow through veins or canals?

Is a canceled check good or void?

Does a window provide a view or a picture?

Is baby beef steak or veal?

Is money safer in your purse or a vault?

Do you put flowers in a shoe or a vase?

Is a car an animal or a vehicle?

Which is a flower, an oak or a violet?

Which is deeper, a valley or a ditch?

Which is worn around the chest, a sock or a vest?

Which is a kind of snake, a beetle or a viper?

Who gets hurt by a crime, the lawyer or the victim?

Was Dracula a vampire or a king?

Which one helps prevent disease, a vaccine or a virus?

The W Sound

We went the wrong _____.	way
He memorized the poem word for _____.	word
The opposite of dry is _____.	wet
North, south, east, and _____.	west
You tell time with a _____.	watch
There's a picture hanging on the _____.	wall
The opposite of cool is _____.	warm
There are seven days in a _____.	week
It is two feet long and three feet _____.	wide
The opposite of tame is _____.	wild
The early bird gets the _____.	worm
Who's afraid of the big, bad _____.	wolf
Toss a penny in the wishing _____.	well
Babies crawl; adults _____.	walk
You dry the dishes and I will _____.	wash
This bird can't fly because it has broken its _____.	wing
My father fought in the Korean _____.	War
The opposite of sick is _____.	well
Before you blow out the candles, make a _____.	wish
I now pronounce you husband and _____.	wife
A word to the _____.	wise
Children play, but adults have to _____.	work
I'd like a glass of ice cold _____.	water
The opposite of man is _____.	woman
It snows in the _____.	winter

151

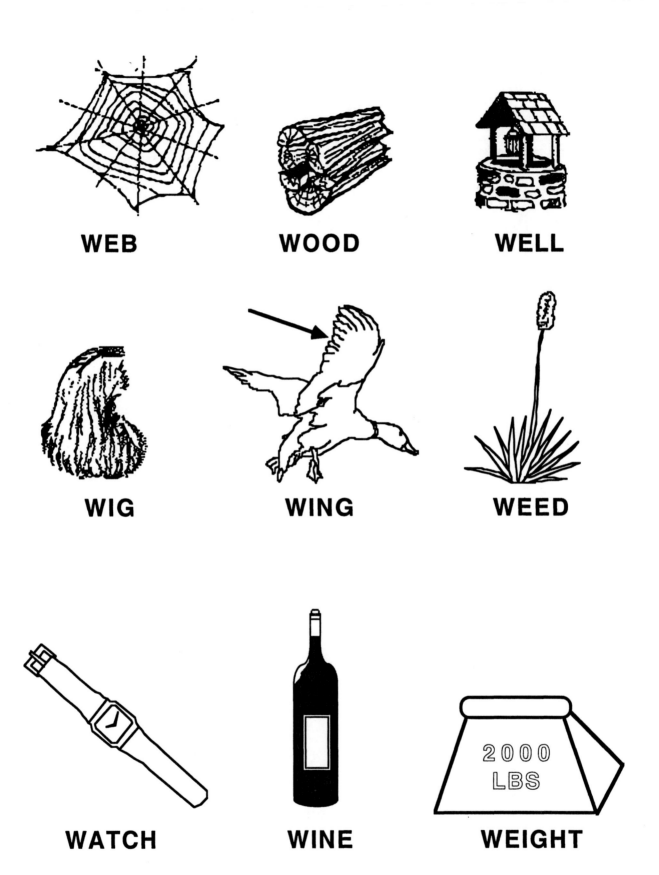

WEB   WOOD   WELL

WIG   WING   WEED

WATCH   WINE   WEIGHT

152

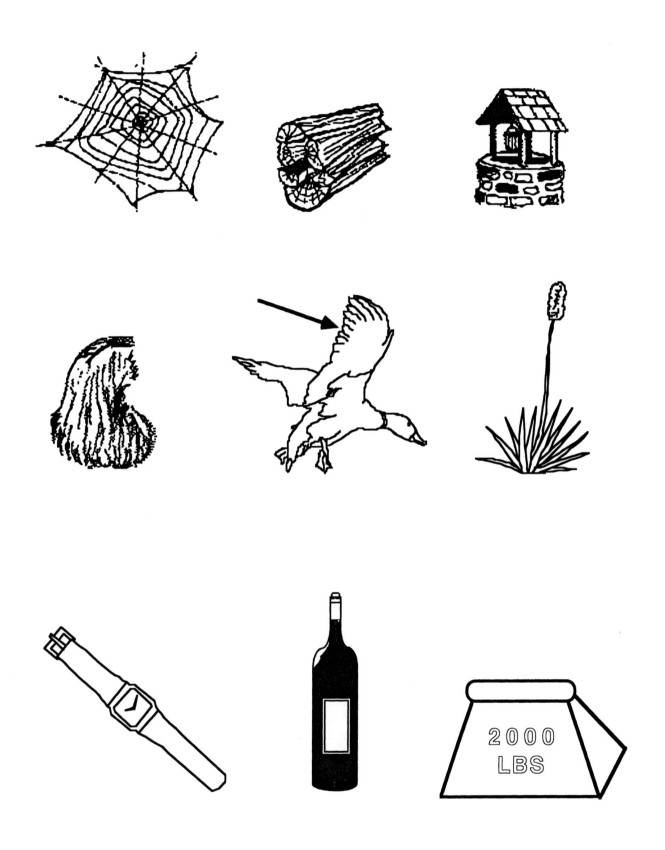

153

we, wee	watt	walk
way, weigh	wet	wand
woe	wit	wind
woo	wing	want
wow	wife	went
weep	wail, wale	ward
wipe	wall	weird
womb	well	word
wine	will, Will	warn
wane, wain, Wayne	wool	worn
win	wire	warp
won	were	wart
wean	war	wasp
web	ware, wear	warm
wake	watch	worm
week, weak	witch	wealth
wick	wash	weld
wag	wish	wild
wig	was	wept
wad	wise	wince
wade	wage	wink
wed	wedge	wolf
weed	wave, waive	worse
wood	weave	worth
wide	with	wound
wait, weight	waist, waste	work
	west	

why

whey

whip

whoop

whim

whine

when

whack

what

wheat

whet

white

whiff

whale

wheel

while

where

which

whoosh

whiz

wheeze

whelp

whence

whirl

whisk

whomp

one-way	want water
we won	well-wisher
we work	wet weather
we will	wash windows
one wife	waterworks
wigwam	water wings
wet wood	waterway
woodwork	wicked witch
woodwind	wishing well
wayward	witty wife
one word	worry wart
walkway	wiggle worm
watchword	welterweight
warm wool	wishy-washy
west wind	welcome wagon
westward	weeping willow
werewolf	winter weather
wormwood	worst world war
well-worn	Will we wait?
wild west	We will wait.
wild wolf	Will we work?
warm wool	We will work.
worst war	Will we wash?
worldwide	We will wash.
world war	We want water.
wall-to-wall	We wash windows.
wash and wear	wild west wagon

We work with words.
We wear warm wool.
Will was wishy-washy.
Willie works with Wanda.
Willie wants a witty wife.
Wanda was a wiggle worm.
The weary washerwoman works well.
The worst war was World War I.

Which is clear, milk or water?

Is California in the east or west?

Does it snow in the winter or the summer?

Which tells time, a watch or a match?

Which is longer, a day or a week?

Is a lion wild or tame?

Do you hang pictures on the wall or the ceiling?

Is it faster to walk or crawl?

Which is deeper, a puddle or a well?

Which will sting, a wasp or a worm?

Does a spider spin a nest or a web?

Is another word for cry, pout or weep?

Is a dandelion a fruit or a weed?

Which is colder, winter or spring?

Do sheep produce cotton or wool?

Which is wilder, a wolf or a dog?

Which is bigger, a woman or a baby?

Which is smaller, a bird or a worm?

Which is alcoholic, water or wine?

Which has wheels, a box or a wagon?

Which looks more like a snake, a bird or a worm?

Which comes from a tree, wood or water?

Which do you need to fly a kite, wind or rain?

Would you rather win or lose?

Is the ocean narrow or wide?

Does a belt go around the wrist or the waist?

NAME ANY EXAMPLE OF A _____.

fruit	meat
vegetable	color
drink	dessert
TV show	drink
room in your house	number
political office	boy's name
part of the body	girl's name
state	jewelry
city	berry
country	job
article of clothing	season
appliance	weather
cooking utensil	building
vehicle	football team
precious gem	shape
kind of dog	food
wild animal	bedding
pet	farm animal
bird	tool
tree	meal
flower	fabric
piece of furniture	instrument
college	religion
sea	river
part of the face	metal
type of shoe	class
type of doctor	floor covering

159

Articulation Therapy Resource for Final Consonant Productions

Final p

bop	cop	pup
beep	cope	pip
chap	coup	pipe
cheap, cheep	cup	wrap
chip	keep	reap
chop	lap	rep
deep	lip	rip
dip	leap	ripe
dope	lop	rope
fop	lope	soap
gap	loop	soup
gape	mope	sop
heap	map	sap
hip	mop	seep
hoop	nap	sip
hop	neap	sup
hope	nip	shape
hype	pop	sheep
jape	poop	ship
jeep	pep	shop
cap	Pope	tap
cape	peep	tape

taupe

tip

top

type

weep

wipe

whip

whoop

Final m

beam	gym, Jim	rim
bomb	gem	rum
boom	jam	roam
bum	cam	room
chime	came	rhyme
chum	comb	seam, seem
dame	come	same
dam	lamb	some, sum
deem	limb	Sam
dim	lame	sham
dime	lime	shame
dome	loom	shim
doom	loam	tam
dumb	ma'am	tame
fame	mom	team
foam	mum	time, thyme
fume	mime	tomb
game	name	tom, Tom
gum	numb	thumb
ham	gnome	vim
him, hymn	Pam	womb
home	ram	whim
hum	ream	

Final n

ban	goon	loin
been, bin	gown	lone, loan
Ben	gone	loon
bone	gain	lawn
bun	gun	lain, lane
bean	hewn	main, mane
chain	hen	men
chin	hone	mine
Dan	gin	moon
den	Jan	mean
dean, Dean	Jane	man
dawn	Jean, gene	moan, mown
dine	John	noun
dune	join	none
down	June	nine
done	can	nun
don, Don	cane	known
deign	con, khan	pain
fan	coin	pan
fawn	cone	pawn
phone	coon	pen
fine	keen	pin
fin	kin	pine
feign, fain	line	pun
fun	lean, lien	pone

ran	ton
reign, rain, rein	town
ruin	tune
run	teen
roan	thin
sane	then
seen, scene	than
soon	thine
sign	van
son, sun	vain, vein, vane
sheen	vine
shin	wine
shine	wain, Wayne
shone, shown	win
shun	won
ten	wean
tin	whine
tine	when

Final b

bib	cube
bob, Bob	lab
babe	lob
dub	lobe
dab	mob
daub	nab
fib	knob
fob	rib
gab	rob
gob	robe
hub	rub
hob	sob
jab	sub
jib	tab
jibe	tube
job	tub
cab	web
cob	

Final k

back	jock	knack
bake	joke	pock
beak	cake	pack
book	cock	peek, peak
buck	coke	peck
check	cook	pike
cheek	kick	pick
chick	kook	poke
choke	lake	rack
chuck	lack	rake
deck	leak, leek	wreck, reck
duke	like	reek
dike	look	rick, Rick
dock, Doc	lick	rock
duck	Luke	rook
fake	lock	sack, sac
gawk	luck	seek
hake	mike, Mike	sake
hack	make	sock
hawk	muck	soak
hick	mock	sick
hike	neck	shack
hock	nick, Nick	shake, sheik
hook	nook	chic, sheik
jack, Jack	knock	shock

shuck

shook

tack

take

tick, tic

took

tuck

wake

week, weak

wick

whack

Final g

bag	log
beg	lug
big	mug
bug	nag
chug	peg, Peg
dug, Doug	pug
dig	pig
dog	rag
fig	rogue
fog	rig
gag	rug
hag	sag
hog	shag
jag	tag
jig	tog
jog	tug
jug	vague
cog	vogue
keg	wag
leg	wig
lag	

Final d

bad	head	mod
bead	had	mood
bed	heed	mud
bid	hid	made, maid
bud	hide	mode
Chad	hod	mead
chide	hood	mid
dude	jade	need, knead
dad	Jude	nod
dead	cad	node
deed	cod	nude
died	code	paid
did	could	pad
dud	cud	pied
fad	kid	pod
fed	lad	raid
feed	laud	read, reed
fade	lead	red, read
feud	load	ride
food	loud	rid
God, god	lid	rude
guide	laid	road, rode
gaud	lewd	rod
goad	led, lead	sad
good	mad	said

seed

side

sod

shad

shade

shed

shod

should

tide

toad

void

wad

wade

wed

weed

wood

wide

Final t

bait	goat	lot
bat	gout	lout
bet	gut	let
beat, beet	hat	mat
bit	hate	mate
bite	heat	meant
bout	height	mint
boot	hit	moat
but, butt	hot	mitt
boat	hoot	might, mite
chit	hut	mutt
cheat	jet	meat, meet
chat	jot	met
dote	jut	mute
date	jute	moot
debt	cat	gnat
dot	coat, cote	not, knot
fat	cot	neat
fate	cut	net
feet, feat	cute	night, knight
fit	kit	knit
fight	kite	note
foot	light	newt
gate, gait	late	naught
get	loot, lute	nut

pat	shoat
pet	shoot, chute
peat, Pete	shot
pit	shout
pot	shut
pout	tot
put	tote
putt	tat
rat	taut, taught
rate	tight
route, rout	tout
right, rite, write	toot
root, route	vat
rot	vet
rote	vote
sat	wait, weight
sit	watt
seat	wet
set	wit
sight, cite, site	what
soot	wheat
sought	whet
suit	white
sheet	

Final ng

bang

ding

dong

fang

gang

hang

hung

king

lung

long

ping

ring, wring

rang

rung, wrung

wrong

sing

sang

sung

song

tong

tongue

wing

173

Final f

buff	life
beef	loaf
chafe	leaf
chaff	luff
chief	laugh
duff	miff
deaf	knife
doff	puff
fife	reef
gaff	rife
goof	roof
guff	rough, ruff
hoof	safe
huff	sheaf
half	chef
Jeff	tiff
calf	tough, tuff
cough	wife
cuff	whiff

Final l

ball, bawl	fool	cull
bail, bale	fell	kale
bell, belle	fuel	keel
bile	gal	kill
bill	gale	loll
boil	gall	lull
bowl	ghoul	mail, male
bull	gill	mall, maul
chill	goal	mile
dale	guile	meal
deal	gull	mill
dial	hail	mole
dill	hall, haul	mull
dole	heel, heal	mule
doll	hill	nail
dull	hull	nil
dell	hole, whole	knell
fail	jail	null
fall	jell, gel	pal
file	Jill	pail, pale
fill, Phil	Joel	pall, Paul
foil	call	peel, peal
full	coal	pile
foul, fowl	coil	pill
feel	cool	pool

poll, pole	tall
pull	teal
rail	tell
reel	tile
rule	till
rile	toil
rill	toll
role, roll	tool
seal	veal
soil	veil, vale
sell	vile
soul, sole	wail
sail, sale	wall
shale	well
shall	will
shawl	wool
shell	whale
shill	wheel
shoal	while
tail, tale	

Final r

bear, bare	jar	roar
bar	jeer	rear
beer	car	rare
bore	care	sear
bur	core	sir
chair	cure	sire
char	leer	soar, sore
cheer	lore	sour
chore	lure	share
dare	lair	shear, sheer
deer, dear	more	shire
dire	mar	shirr
door	mare	shore
for, four, fore	mire	tar
fir, fur	moor	tear
fire	mere	tare, tear
far	nor	tire
fair, fare	near	tour
fear	par	veer
gar	pair, pare, pear	wire
gear	peer, pier	were
hair, hare	pure	war
hire, higher	pore, pour	ware, wear
here, hear	poor	where

Final s

base, bass	hiss	muss
bass	jess, Jess	moose
bus	juice	mace
boss	case	moss
chase	cuss	niece
chess	kiss	nice
choice	lass	noose
deuce	lace	pace
dice	less	pass
dose	lice	peace, piece
douse, dowse	loss	rice
dace	louse	race
face	lease	sass
fuss	loose	sis
gas	mice	sauce
guess	mass	toss
geese	miss	vase
goose	mouse	vice, vise
house	mess	voice

Final ch

beach, beech
church
hooch
coach
leach, leech
loach
mooch
much
peach
poach
reach
rich
roach
such
teach
touch
vouch
watch
witch
which

Final sh

bush	lush
bash	mash
dish	mesh
dash	mush
fish	gnash
gash	posh
gosh	push
gush	rash
hush	rush
hash	sash
josh, Josh	shush
cash	wash
leash	wish
lash	whoosh

Final z

buzz	laze
booze	maze, maize
cheese	muse
chose	news
choose	nose
doze	noise
daze	pose
does	poise
faze, phase	pause
fuzz	raise
fuse	razz
fizz	rise
gaze	rose, rows
gauze	rouse
guise, guys	size
haze	seize
hose	wise
jazz	was
cause	whiz
lose	wheeze

Final v

chive	move
dove	mauve
dive	knave
five	pave
gave	peeve
give	rave
have	reeve
heave	rove
hove	rive
hive	save
jive	sieve
cave	shave
cove	shove
live	sheave
leave	wave, waive
love	weave

Final j

beige
gauge
gouge
huge
judge
cage
page
rage
rouge
sage
siege
wedge
wage

183

Final Voiceless th

bath
Beth
both
booth
death
faith
heath
kith
lath
math
moth
myth
mouth
path
with
wrath
south
sheath
teeth
tooth

Final Voiced th

bathe
loathe
lathe
seethe
soothe

185

BUTTERWORTH-HEINEMANN ORDER FORM

FOUR WAYS TO ORDER!

1.	2.	3.	4.
Call us toll-free at: **800-366-2665** Monday - Friday, 8:00AM - 6:00PM Eastern Time.	**Mail your order to:** **Butterworth-Heinemann Fulfillment Center 225 Wildwood Ave. Woburn, MA 01801**	**E-Mail your order to:** orders@repp.com	**Fax your order toll-free to:** **800-446-6520**

Please send me the following:

Quantity   Title/Author/ISBN   Price

_____   *Take Time to Talk, 2/e*, White, 0-7506-9783-0, $25.00 ea. _____   _____

_____   _____   _____

_____   _____   _____

_____   _____   _____

                                               Subtotal   _____

                     Your state sales tax   _____

                               Handling*   _____

❑ I have enclosed a check for $ _____   *   TOTAL   _____
(Submit in U.S. Funds, payable to Butterworth-Heinemann. U.S. residents please include state sales tax.)

Please charge my:

     ❑ Visa   ❑ MasterCard   ❑ American Express

Card no. _____ Exp. date _____

Cardholder name _____

Signature _____
                  (Signature required on all orders.)

❑ Bill me*   ❑ Bill my institution: PO no. _____

Name _____

Institution _____
          (please give street address. We cannot deliver to PO Boxes)

Address _____

City_____ State ____ Zip _____

Phone (_____) _____

* Please add $4.00 handling fee for the first item ordered, $1.50 for each additional item, to all check and credit card orders. Billed orders will be charged additional shipping based on weight and destination. All U.S. orders must include your state sales tax. Prices subject to change without notice.

Canadian Customers: please pay by credit card or in U.S. funds and include 7% GST on books and handling.

NO RISK! 30-DAY
EXAMINATION PERIOD!
Order your 30-day approval copies today! We believe you'll find them valuable clinical references. If not, simply return them and we will cancel your invoice or issue a refund.

Q42